THE

MW01593938

50 YEARS OF LEADERSHIP: CONTINUING THE VISION

CELEBRATING 50 YEARS OF THE COMMUNICATING NURSING RESEARCH CONFERENCE

and

60TH ANNIVERSARY OF THE WESTERN COUNCIL ON HIGHER EDUCATION FOR NURSING (WCHEN) / THE WESTERN INSTITUTE OF NURSING (WIN)

The Western Institute of Nursing is indebted to Elaine S. Marshall, PhD, RN, FAAN, who, with colleagues, created the 50th Communicating Nursing Research conference anniversary book. The history of this trailblazing conference cannot be told without the story of the 60th anniversary of the Western Council on Higher Education for Nursing (WCHEN) / Western Institute of Nursing (WIN), which originated and continues to offer this landmark conference. WCHEN/WIN was founded on this principle: nursing research, education and the improvement of patient care are highly interrelated. This principle endures today and into the future. Finally, the Anniversary Book tells the story of the strong leaders who originated the organization and conference. We stand on the shoulders of these Western giants.

WESTERN INSTITUTE OF NURSING
SN-4S
3455 SW US VETERANS HOSPITAL ROAD
PORTLAND, OR 97239-2941

An Affirmative Action/Equal Opportunity Employer

Spring 2017

TABLE OF CONTENTS

PREFACE

In *The Winds of Change,* Pearl Coulter was compelled to tell the "the history of half a decade" of the Western Council on Higher Education for Nursing (WCHEN), saying, "Nursing educators in the West are committed to a belief that the future can be greater than the past if the sails are properly trimmed and the outmoded aspects of the past and present are cast overboard" (Coulter, 1963, p. 1). She further noted:

> Here is a story of activities which could have taken place only under a specific set of circumstances . . . activities growing out of a conviction that the people of the West need nursing services of excellent quality and that nursing education must prepare people capable of providing that service . . . busy people who were willing to extend themselves even further because they saw needs that were inadequately met (Coulter, 1963, p. 2).

We now tell the story of half a century of *Communicating Nursing Research.* The story is no less compelling than Coulter's observations. To tell the story of a conference is a daunting task. To simply review the themes or statistics related to each meeting would be an unfortunate exercise that would overlook the very life of the conference. A conference, especially one that has vibrantly endured for 50 years, is, by definition, a gathering of people. Conferences are made by the people who dream and envision, plan, execute, share, participate, and interpret their experiences to make a better world. This conference, *Communicating Nursing Research,* began as a dream of bold leaders who were pioneers in the West in every sense of the word. It has continued with the commitment of stellar leaders who have given from their best intellectual brains and devoted hearts. Each person who has participated in these conferences in any way has his or her own story. These stories need to be shared to build on moving to the next 50 years.

Coulter also proclaimed, "This story could be, with good reason, a collection of biographical episodes in the lives of a group of nurse educators" (Coulter, 1963, p. 2). This is a story about people, important people with courage and vision. Wherever a name appeared in the archival documents, I wanted to know more about this person. Who was he or she? What was the experience of his or her life? Wherever possible, I have expanded on the story of the person so that readers might become better acquainted with the actual people who created our story. Of course, especially as the conference grew to its amazing number of participants, it was not possible to describe or even include all the folks who made such a difference. For that, I regret that I was not able to share the lives of so many who gave so much.

My adventure through the last 50 years of the *Communicating Nursing Research* conference, the first of its kind and model for other regions in the country, has confirmed my belief that it is the pioneers of the West who most dared to risk innovation. They altruistically broke new paths so that those who followed would have a better way. They actively engaged to get the work done, found resources to support the work, and collaborated. They were bold with their own ideas tempered with a willingness to listen those of others.

It is clear that this is a celebratory history, and thus written in a more positive than analytic tone. But I have endeavored to lay out the events and tell the stories of the people in a way that you may add your own analysis and your own story.

Elaine Sorensen Marshall, PhD, RN, FAAN

ACKNOWLEDGEMENTS

What an honor and amazing fun it has been to explore and report the story of the first 50 years of the Western Institute of Nursing (WIN) *Communicating Nursing Research* conference. Much of the pleasure has come from the people who have given their time, interest, memories, skills, and love to this project.

Special thanks to Paula McNeil for her many efforts to keep this organization going. There is nothing she hasn't agreed to do to support this project—far beyond the expectations of her already highly demanding work at WIN. Thanks also to Laura Hottman at the WIN headquarters.

Thanks to the members of the History Subcommittee for this 50th Celebration of the conference. Without their generosity to help conceptualize, plan, read drafts, correct, and lend their first-hand memories of events, this work could not have been done. I am their deepest admirer and they are forever friends to WIN:
Marjorie Batey
Jeanne Kearns
Carol Lindeman
Elizabeth Nichols

Thanks to the members of the History Celebration Planning Committee for their support:
Martha Lentz, Chair
Marjorie Batey
Denise Bartley
Bonnie Gance-Cleveland
Linda Gregory
Jeanne Kearns
Marie Lobo
Laura Perry
Michael Rice

Special thanks to nurse historian colleagues. They shared the vision, dug into dusty archives, enriched the story, and saved the day:

Barbara Gaines - for finding treasures, asking the right questions, expanding my thinking, and helping with the writing. Much of Chapter 6 is in Barbara's words;

Brigid Lusk - for responding with just the right data at just the right time; and

Jane Lassetter – for providing, on a moment's notice, just the resources needed.

Thanks to my husband, John; my children; and my dear friends who supported me with patience and cheers to the finish line to complete the project.

Elaine Sorensen Marshall, PhD, RN, FAAN

Chapter One

THE WORK BEGINS: 1951-1968

Chapter One
THE WORK BEGINS: 1951-1968

The Western Institute of Nursing (WIN), with its distinguished annual *Communicating Nursing Research* conference, began with the vision of a few pioneers of an organization to improve health care by advancing professional nursing in higher education across the Western region of the United States. Such an ambitious plan for regional collaboration was among the first in the United States, and its annual conference was indeed the first of its kind and continues to be the oldest in the country (WIN, 2016a). From the beginning, the importance of a shared journey to raise the level of education and research in the region was path-breaking. An important theme throughout the history of WIN is the impressive contributions of some of the finest leaders in nursing in the United States whose devotion to the discipline in the Western region helped to establish WIN's continuing reputation in higher education and research.

Madeleine Leininger (1992, p. 43) noted that WCHEN [the Western Council on Higher Education for Nursing and forerunner of WIN] was:

> . . . a unique and innovative organizational structure and a model in America and for the world to advance nursing education and practice. It was a cadre of wise and spirited nurse leaders who had great vision and plans to make nursing a distinct discipline and an important example to the public and nursing organizations.

In 1951, the Western Interstate Commission on Higher Education (WICHE) was created by governors and legislators of 13 Western states (WIN, 1992, p. 9; see Note 1-A). The compact was created to facilitate regional cooperation to share resources related to all aspects of higher education among the states. It officially began in 1953 with headquarters in Eugene, Oregon and moved to its current location in Boulder, Colorado in 1955. It has functioned under commissioners appointed by Western governors and through annual dues from each member state. It currently includes 15 states and the Northern Mariana Islands (WICHE, 2016) (See Note 1-B).

First Director of WICHE: Harold Enarson
The first Executive Director, Harold Enarson, set the precedent for outstanding leadership of the organization. He was born on a farm near the small town of Villisca, Iowa. Soon, his family moved to New Mexico, where he grew up during the Great Depression. After the Japanese attack on Pearl Harbor, he enlisted in the Army and earned several medals, including the Purple Heart for wounds acquired while serving in Germany (Find a Grave, 2010). He graduated from the University of New Mexico and later became the first president of Cleveland State University (Associated Press, 2006). He was President of The Ohio State University, where he was known for the brave, controversial firing of the well-known football coach, Woody Hayes, following an unfortunate incident against an opposing player for which the coach apparently refused to apologize. The capstone of Enarson's distinguished career was his return to the West for his service of 20 years as Director and advisor for WICHE (Associated Press, 2006).

As early as 1954, nursing issues in higher education were among the most important issues discussed by WICHE Commissioners (WIN, 1992; 2007). By 1955, Enarson called for a group of professionals to advise the WICHE Commission on issues related to nursing education in the West. Thus, Vera Fry, professor of public health nursing at the University of California Berkeley, was appointed to lead the *Western Regional Meeting on Advanced Education for Nursing*, held in St. Louis prior to the convention of the National League of Nursing (NLN). With a focus on the need for graduate education in nursing, the purpose of the meeting was to address "broad principles, curricula, finances, best utilization of finances, best utilization of faculty and others" (WIN, 1992, p. 9).

Vera Fry brought at least a decade of experience in graduate education and nursing. She was named Director of Nursing Education Curriculum at New York University (NYU) in 1944. She established the Department of Nursing at NYU in 1947 and served as its founding leader until the arrival of the famed leader and theorist, Martha E. Rogers, in 1954 (NYU College of Nursing, 2016; NYU Rory Meyers College of Nursing, 2016). Fry is also credited to have been the first to introduce the concept of "nursing diagnosis" to the profession (Fry, 1953; See Dunphy, 2009).

With Fry, Enarson convened an interim advisory committee to push forward the agenda toward increasing opportunities for high-quality graduate education in nursing across the West. The committee recommended that NLN provide a consultant to WICHE (WIN, 1992, p. 9).

Helen Nahm fit the requirements. Educated in Missouri and Minnesota, she had served as Director of the University of Missouri School of Nursing, Director of the Division of Nursing at Duke University, and had served as Director of the National Nursing Accrediting Service and Director of the Department of Baccalaureate and Higher Degree Programs at NLN from 1952 to 1953. By 1955, when she agreed to consult with WICHE, she was Director of the Division of Nursing Education at NLN. Nahm was known as a distinguished thinker in the profession. Throughout her career, she articulated an "explicit difference between medicine and nursing," and envisioned nursing as an independent practice profession (Mirsky, Olesen, & Weiss, 1992, p. 128). Following her work with WICHE, she served as the dean of the School of Nursing at the University of California San Francisco from 1958 to 1969, where she established one of the first doctoral programs in nursing and created one of the first basic science departments within a school of nursing. She served as Chair of WCHEN in 1961 (See Mirsky, et al., 1992; "Online archive," 2016; Schwartz, 2014; UCSF, 2016; WIN, 2016b).

The Nahm Report and the Berkeley Conference
Nahm surveyed the schools of nursing in the West with aspirations to develop graduate curricula from a perspective of "cooperative" and "imaginative approaches to graduate training in nursing" (WIN, 1992, p. 9). By 1956, her report was ready to share at the next WICHE conference on nursing.

Nahm had visited 20 of the 33 colleges and universities in the region that offered programs in nursing. At the time, there were no collegiate schools of nursing in four of the Western states: Alaska, Arizona, New Mexico, and Nevada. Only six institutions offered master's degrees in nursing: University of California Berkeley; University of

California Los Angeles; College of Medical Evangelists, Loma Linda, CA; University of Colorado, Boulder; University of Oregon, Portland; and University of Washington in Seattle. There were no doctoral programs in nursing in the region, and only about ten nurse faculty members actually held doctoral degrees. Of the 9,814 students enrolled in nursing programs in the West, 28 percent were in collegiate schools of nursing, with the rest in hospital diploma programs (Nahm, 1956).

Nahm outlined extensive observations and reports from Western institutions of higher education and schools of nursing. Most of her report offered evidence to document the need for "better prepared administrators and supervisors in nursing service agencies, both hospital and public health, for better prepared administrators in schools of nursing . . . and for nurses who are prepared to design, conduct, and supervise research in nursing" (Nahm, 1956, p. 47). The general theme of Nahm's data-rich report was the need across the region to improve access to and prevalence of opportunities for higher education for nurses, with a focus on the need for graduate preparation of nurses in leadership, teaching, and research roles. The report confirmed a need for approaches to resolve such issues at the regional, inter-state level, thus confirming the vision of a Western regional organization of nurses.

In 1956, WICHE convened the conference *Toward Shared Planning in Western Nursing Education* in Berkeley California, and the Nahm report was shared. This became known to WICHE and WIN historians as "The Berkeley Conference" (Coulter, 1963; WIN, 2007, p. 39). Participants recommended the formation of a committee, "of not more than seven members," to plan for the establishment of a Western Council on Higher Education for Nursing (WCHEN) and an annual regional conference (WIN, 1992, p. 9). Following the recommendations, Enarson immediately appointed what became known as the first "Committee of Seven" to begin the work.

The Committee of Seven
Members of the first Committee of Seven were Lulu Hassenplug, Chair; Pearl Coulter, James Enochs, Katherine Hoffman, Annette Lefkowitz, Amelia Leino, and Kathryn Smith. Who were these seven members of this illustrious group?

Lulu Hassenplug held degrees from the Army School of Nursing at Walter Reed Hospital, Columbia University, and Johns Hopkins University. She served as a faculty member at Vanderbilt University School of Nursing (Oliver, 1995; Shipley, 1980). She was the founding dean of the School of Nursing at the University of California Los Angeles (UCLA), serving from 1949 to 1968, and designated *Woman of the Year* in 1958 by the *Los Angeles Times.* She was a strong proponent of moving nursing education from the hospital to the university campus, remembered as saying, "We are training nurses to think. This is the purpose of a liberal education. A well-trained mind can usually handle any difficulty. A well-trained mind is basic to giving individualized patient care" (Oliver, 1995). She served as Chair of WCHEN in 1964 (WIN, 2016b).

Pearl Parvin Coulter was born in Almyra, Arkansas and studied at Kansas Wesleyan College and the University of Colorado. She trained in public health and nursing at George Peabody College in Nashville, Tennessee and Yale University in Connecticut. Before coming to Colorado, she was Director of public health in the School of Nursing at the University of Wisconsin. She was a professor in the School of Nursing at the University of Colorado for 10 years before becoming the first female dean and the founding dean of the University of Arizona College of Nursing in 1957 (Denogean, 2002; Humphrey, 2002; University of Arizona, 2002). She advanced the idea that nurses should be educated in an academic institution, "using the hospital as a laboratory for educational purposes," (Humphrey, 2002) while promoting strong collaboration between nursing education and practice (Denogean, 2002). She also envisioned graduate education at the doctoral level for nurses, and she lived to see the achievement of the doctor of philosophy (Ph.D.) degree implemented at Arizona shortly after her retirement (Humphrey, 2002). Devoted to WCHEN, Coulter wrote its first significant history, *The Winds of Change,* in 1963.

James B. Enochs was a highly-respected administrator and expert on higher education in the state of California. He was born in Hayden, Colorado and spent his early years in several states in the west, including New Mexico and Montana as his father's employment required family moves. He attended the University of Mississippi and earned the Ph.D. from the University of Chicago (S. T. Enochs, personal communication, February 1, 2017). He represented the California State Department of Education on a "Restudy Staff" commissioned in 1955 to examine the needs of the state in higher education (McConnell, Holy, & Semans, 1955). He was the first Dean of Academic Planning for the California State Colleges, working in the Chancellor's office. This was a critical time of transition of the state colleges from the general status of teacher's colleges to become part of "an integrated Master Plan covering all of higher education in California" and eventually to become state universities. His expertise was in curriculum development, and he helped to develop curricular changes in nursing education, social work programs, engineering education, and agricultural education. He served on the California State Master Plan Committee until 1962. While he consulted on higher education curriculum development across the country, he served as Dean of Graduate Study at Los Angeles State College (WCHEN, 1961). In 1963, he moved to the new two-year-old Sonoma State University (see SSU, 2016), where he helped to establish the nursing department and eventually became University Executive Vice President (S. T. Enochs, personal communication, February 1, 2017). There, he continued to focus on strengthening graduate programs and the nursing program (Anderson, 1975; James Enochs Papers, 1999). He worked in the California State College system for 27 years (Anderson, 1975). Following his service on the first Committee of Seven, he continued to support activities of nursing programs at WICHE. For example, he was noted on the program as a speaker at WCHEN's annual conferences in 1958 and 1961 (WCHEN, 1958a; 1961). He retired in 1975 and moved to Ashland, Oregon (Anderson, 1975), where he and his wife, Elizabeth (Terry) were active in church and community organizations, including usher at the local theater. Dr. Enochs died in 1993 (S. T. Enochs, personal communication February 1, 2017).

Katherine Hoffman was born in Grand Forks, British Columbia and graduated from Tacoma General Hospital School of Nursing in 1934. She is known as the first nurse in the state of Washington to earn the Doctor of Philosophy (in 1956). She was a faculty member at the University of Washington, and committed to the advancement of graduate education and research in nursing, serving as Director of graduate programs, Assistant Dean, and Assistant Dean for the university's Health Sciences Division (M. V. Batey, personal communication, August 16, 2016). She was a charter member of the American Academy of Nursing (ANA, 2016; WSNA, 1996, 2004).

Annette S. Lefkowitz grew up in Pennsylvania (A. Lefkowitz to B. Lusk, personal communication, n. d., NIU SON archives) and graduated from New York Hospital-Cornell Medical School of Nursing in 1941. She earned the B.A. from Pennsylvania State University (Penn State) in 1949, and the M.A. and Ed.D. degrees from Teacher's College of Columbia University in New York in 1954 and 1958 respectively. Her dissertation was a history of the nursing program at Idaho State College/University in Pocatello (A. Lefkowitz to B. Lusk, n. d.). She began her career as a staff nurse at New York Hospital, joined the Army Nurse Corps and served in the Philippines, then returned to school under the GI Bill in Pennsylvania (A. Lefkowitz to B. Lusk, n. d.). While there, from 1946 to 1953, she was a dormitory nurse at Penn State and instructor and subsequent Director of the School of Nursing and Director of Nursing Services at Lock Haven Hospital in Lock Haven, Pennsylvania. In 1954, she came West as Director of the Department of Nursing at Idaho State College in Pocatello where she became active in WCHEN. She left the West in 1958 as consultant and founded the School of Nursing at Northern Illinois University in 1959 (NLN record, 1971). She led the school until 1978 and continued as professor until 1985 (A. Lefkowitz, letter to Dean Peggy Sullivan, June 18, 1984, NIU SON archives; Marsh, 1969; "Northern Illinois School," 2009). A research fund in her name continues at the University (College of Health & Human Sciences, 2007). She died in 2001 at the age of 79 in Fort Myers, Florida and is buried in her home town of Shenandoah, Pennsylvania (*News-Press*, 2001).

Amelia Leino was born in Three Town, and grew up in Hanna, Wyoming, where she was a star high school basketball player. She left her tiny western coal mining town for Chicago where she graduated from nursing school at Cook County Hospital. She later joined the United States Army Nurse Corps during World War II, and eventually completed graduate degrees at Teachers College at Columbia University. In 1951, she returned to her home state to become the first woman dean and the founding dean of the School of Nursing at the University of Wyoming where she served until 1968. She was devoted to the work of WICHE and influenced the establishment of the first chapter of Sigma Theta Tau International in the state of Wyoming (Anderson, 2015; University of Wyoming, 2001).

Kathryn Smith (Lastreto) was born in Flandreau, South Dakota; graduated in nursing from the University of Minnesota, and earned the Ed.D. from Stanford University (Napa Valley Register, 2004). At the time of her service on the Committee of Seven, she was a faculty member at the School of Nursing at the University of California Medical Center in San Francisco (Smith, 1956). She was Dean of the School of Nursing at the University of Colorado at Denver from 1965 to 1974, the first with doctoral preparation. In 1967, she was nominated by President Lyndon Johnson as the first woman member of the board of regents of the National Library of Medicine. She also served for 17 years as Assistant Dean of the University of California Los Angeles School of Nursing, and as a Commissioner of WICHE (CU, 2005; Napa Valley Register, 2004; WICHE, 1969). She was elected Chair of WCHEN 1969-1970 (WIN, 2016b). She passed away on March 17, 2004.

Most of these founding leaders pursued their commitments to WICHE, WCHEN, and WIN throughout their lives. For their continued service, the following were eventually the first to be awarded Emerita status of the Western Institute of Nursing: Lulu Hassenplug, Pearl Parvin Coulter, Katherine Hoffman, Kathryn Smith Lastreto, and Amelia Leino (WIN, 2016c). The names of Harold Enarson and Helen Nahm were also later added to the distinguished Emeriti list.

The Committee of Seven met in Denver, March 5-8, 1956 with consultants Helen Nahm and Marion Sheahan from NLN, Margaret Arnstein from the United States Public Health Service, and Margaret Taylor from the University of California, Los Angeles (Coulter, 1963). High anticipation of the significance of the Committee decisions and recommendations are evident in Coulter's own words:

> It [was] rumored that Dr. Enarson locked the group in a small hotel room in Denver, put the key in his pocket, and shouted through the keyhole, "You may come out when you have produced an imaginative, creative program." On the other hand, weather reports show than nature contrived a blizzard into which only the most robust would dare venture . . . whether because of administrative direction, the raging storm, inherent individual drive, or the dynamics of the group, they *did* stay in that hotel, took their assignment seriously, and produced a plan of action! *It is upon the specific design developed by the Committee that the subsequent structure and program of the Western Council on Higher Education for Nursing* [and eventually the Western Institute of Nursing] *has been built* (Coulter, 1963, p. 16).

The Committee divided itself into sub-committees on Organization, Doctoral Programs, Continuing Education, and Research with all coming together on final recommendations. Coulter outlined in detail the recommendations, objectives, functions, that successfully launched WCHEN (see Coulter, 1963). Specifically related to research, Coulter (1963, p. 18) summarized the report of the Research Sub-Committee:

> Nurses are eager to assume their responsibility for directing research studies in nursing. They are now asking for educational opportunities that will prepare them to meet their obligations to society . . . Research is needed to identify the factors contributing to the nursing needs of patients and families in hospitals and community services . . . The greatest single obstacle in going forward in research in nursing is the lack of nurses with preparation to do research.

In those four short days in March, 1956, the Committee of Seven prepared a 30-page report that "included recommendations on the organizational structure of a Western Council on Higher Education for Nursing [WCHEN], as well as a plan of action on three fronts: continuing education, development of doctoral level programs, and fellowships for graduate study in nursing" (Coulter, 1963, p. 20). Coulter (1963, p. 20) reflected, "The report of the Committee of Seven was, in essence, a synthesis of the dreams and hopes of nursing leaders in the Western region . . ."

Support and Leadership for the New Organization
It was clear that WICHE would not be able to fund all of the ambitious recommendations of the Committee of Seven. Leaders and staff of WICHE immediately prepared a proposal for distribution to potential funding sources entitled *Professional Training for Western Nurses: A Plan of Action.* The document included statements on WICHE's interest and support, a review of the Berkeley Conference, and the report of the Committee of Seven (Coulter, 1963, p. 21). The W. K. Kellogg Foundation responded, providing support for a nurse consultant for the first five years and a continuing education project for its first three years. So, Faye Abdellah joined the WICHE staff as the nurse consultant (Coulter, 1963, WIN, 1992; WIN, 2007).

Abdellah was the Chief of the Education Branch of the United States Public Health Service. Her primary role was to establish WCHEN's continuing education initiatives. She graduated from Ann May School of Nursing (renamed Raleigh Fitkin-Paul Morgan Memorial Hospital) (Jersey Shore University Medical Center, 2016), and earned baccalaureate, masters, and doctoral degrees from Columbia University. Her tenure at WICHE was brief but significant, and the enthusiastic response and support among state nursing leaders are credited to her efforts. She eventually became one of the most respected leaders in nursing. She was the first nurse officer to receive the rank of a two-star admiral, the first nurse and first woman to serve as Deputy Surgeon General, and she founded the Graduate School of Nursing at the Uniformed Services University of the Health Sciences and served as its first dean (ANA, 2012; Jersey Shore University Medical Center, 2016; National Women's Hall of Fame, 2016). She became best known for her work promoting research and as a nurse theorist for her work on "Twenty-one Nursing Problems" and patient-centered, rather than disease-focused approach to nursing (See Abdellah, Beland, Martin, & Matheney, 1960; Abdellah & Levine, 1965). Dr. Abdellah died on February 24, 2017 at the age of 97.

Within a few short months, leaders came together in a remarkable unity of vision toward the future of nursing in the West. These leaders were strong, competitive, individuals with impressive backgrounds in experience and training. They volunteered extraordinary time and effort, were willing to move in uncharted professional territory, and each held a significant "day job" in his or her own local sphere. They understood organization and offered an entrepreneurial spirit (many were or became founding deans, and often the first female deans in their institution). They also understood the importance of financial support and sought funding for organization from the beginning. Historical evidence is silent on any significant professional protection of territory or interest in personal gain among these strong professional pioneers. Disagreement, or dissent that might be expected are assumed to have erupted to some degree along the way and emerge among anecdotal memories, but are remarkably rarely noted. The efforts of these leaders were historic, not only in formulating a new visionary organization, but in the uncommon willingness to collaborate across institutional and state boundaries toward betterment of developing profession throughout a very large geographic region and subsequent improvement of societal well-being. Such professional altruism is noteworthy. Indeed, Coulter quoted the following message from Harold Enarson, himself:

> . . . In your candid appraisal of the status of Western nursing education, we think you are exhibiting one of the most important qualities of a profession: the capacity of critical introspection . . . We think the possibilities of inter-school cooperation across state lines is a frontier of unexplored opportunity (Coulter, 1963, p. 24).

The First Organizational Meeting
The first meeting of WCHEN, held on the campus of San Francisco State College on January 30-31, 1957, included more than 50 representatives of baccalaureate and graduate programs in nursing from throughout the West. Participants had received the proposed charter of the organization in advance of the meeting, so they came ready for discussion and debate.

Three specific areas, "points of anxiety" (Coulter, 1963, p. 24) regarding membership, were ultimately resolved. First, since a major purpose of the organization was a focus on graduate education, there was some question on eligibility of schools with baccalaureate programs only, whose leaders were anxious to participate. It was resolved that such programs would be eligible for membership, since the baccalaureate degree graduates fed into graduate programs.

This led to the second issue, which related to representation and control on the Council. Since the number of baccalaureate programs far outweighed the number of graduate programs in the region, it was decided that each institution with both undergraduate and graduate programs in nursing would be allowed four representatives; schools with graduate programs only would have three representatives; and those offering the baccalaureate only would have one representative (Coulter, 1963).

The third concern was "fear of domination" by a single state. This was largely directed at California, due to the rapid development of the California State College group. Though the Committee of Seven had suggested "collective representation" for the entire group, "democracy triumphed over fear, and each school was assured its fair voice and vote in the Council" (Coulter, 1963, p. 24).

Participants agreed that membership would be open to accredited institutions in the region with programs in nursing leading to baccalaureate or higher degrees (see Note 1-C). The Council would meet semi-annually, and four Seminar groups would be established: Continuing Education, Undergraduate Education, Graduation Education, and Research. The charter of the Council established the following functions:

1. Recommend to the Commission policies relating to graduate education and research in nursing.

2. Provide a medium for the exchange of ideas and the sharing of experiences of the individual Western institutions of higher learning which offer programs of education for professional nursing.

3. Undertake cooperative planning for nursing educational programs within the Western region under the auspices of the Commission.

4. Identify problems with respect to nursing education which need cooperative study.

5. Stimulate research in nursing within the colleges and universities of the Western region (Coulter, 1963, p. 25; WCHEN, 1957, p. 63; WIN, 1992, p. 10).

WCHEN is Launched

To become effective as an official inter-institutional and inter-state organization, assent was required from a majority of eligible institutions. The first vote was signed and sent by the president of the University of Hawaii (Coulter, 1963; WIN, 1992). By the end of 1957, thirty-one institutions across the 13 states of the West had joined (Coulter, 1963).

The Pioneer Leader of WCHEN: Jo Eleanor Elliott

By July 1957, Jo Eleanor Elliott interrupted graduate study to replace Abdellah as the permanent nurse consultant at WICHE. She was born in LaMonte, Missouri, attended Central Missouri State College, and earned the baccalaureate in nursing from the University of Michigan and eventually a master's degree from the University of Chicago. She held faculty positions at the University of Michigan and the University of California Los Angeles (Bak, 2011; Cipriano, 2011; Culver, 2011; Curtin, 2011; Denver Post, 2011; "Jo Eleanor Elliott," 1980; Sachs, 2011; WIN, 2016c). Elliott led WCHEN for 23 years: from 1957 until 1980.

In 1959, Elliott produced an impressive, bold, and comprehensive report on the current and projected future issues and needs related to nursing in the West. She challenged leaders at the local, regional, and institutional level to increase nursing graduates and education levels to meet the needs for the next 11 years. For example, drawing from evidence from each state in the region, she outlined projected needs to expand graduates from master's and post-master's programs from the then current 125 per year to over 1,000 per year in the region (see Elliott, 1959, p. 38). A follow-up report in 1966 confirmed the need to continue to prepare nurses for the region, including efforts at research by nurses (see Pair, 1966).

In 1963, Elliott was one of eight nurse leaders honored at the Presidio in San Francisco by the commanding officer of the Sixth U. S. Army Recruiting District (Abbott, 2004, p. 96—see Note 1-E). While continuing to lead WCHEN, from 1964 to 1968, Elliott also served as President of the American Nurses Association (ANA), leading the organization as one of the initial and consistent supporters of the Medicare act. She was present when President Lyndon B. Johnson signed the act into law as well as the Nurse Training Act to Aid Professional Nurse Education. In 1966, as she led the ANA convention delegates to debate the controversial position to recommend a baccalaureate degree in nursing as the minimum preparation for a professional nurse, her words offer wisdom for any issue and time. She said:

> It is a monumental complicated, lengthy task to move from a statement of position to the effecting of change through orderly transition. No such change can be carried out without the full participation of nurses at every level . . . No such change can come about merely because nurses will it to occur . . . No such change begins in this moment of time . . . Change will occur anyway. Our task is to see that it is orderly, not chaotic—planned change rather than change that has been allowed to just happen" (Elliott, 1966, p. 1554).

Her leadership skills, command of the issues in nursing education and practice, her tireless devotion to effective support and communication among nursing and academic leaders across the West, and her own personal charisma established the strong a foundation for the organization. She was beloved and known to be "fearless and high-spirited" (Bak, 2011). In 1968, she launched the first annual *Communicating Nursing Research Conference*.

Following her service to WCHEN, Elliott became the Director of the Division of Nursing for the United States Public Health Services until 1989. In 1988, Jeanne Kearns, a successor at WCHEN, established the Jo Eleanor Elliott Leadership Award, which has now honored 24 nursing leaders in the West (WIN, 2016c).

In 2010, upon passage of health care reform, President Barack Obama praised Elliott for "the courage and leadership she showed" for her lifelong work to improve

American health care. That same year, when honored with the "President's Award as a Champion for Nursing Education" by NLN, her response was, "Helmets down, lances up, full speed ahead" (Bak, 2011).

After the death of Jo Eleanor Elliott in 2011, Thelma Schorr, former editor of the American Journal of Nursing, recalled "She was a visionary and stood firm" (Culver, 2011). Leah Curtin noted her "uncommon" common sense, her "wit and wisdom:" "Nothing about Jo Eleanor was common—she was an extraordinary leader . . . I wish there was some way we could make people like her available to students. If we did, there would be no more lamenting our lack of leadership!" (Curtin, 2011).

Under the leadership of Elliott, the visions of the pioneer leaders and the functions of the original charter of WCHEN became vibrant realities. A daunting number of successful projects on all aspects of nursing education was initiated, including an annual regional conference on issues in nursing, specific projects, including the following examples: *Continuing Education in Leadership, Defining Clinical Content: Graduate Nursing Programs, Identification of Essential Content in Baccalaureate Programs in Nursing, Developing a Q-Sort Instrument to Delineate Differences Between Graduates of Baccalaureate and Associate Degree Programs, and Curriculum Improvement,* as well as surveys of nursing needs and resources, seminars on junior college nursing programs, staff development, improving instruction, undergraduate nursing program issues, inclusion of representation of associate degree nursing programs, and the annual conference.

Elliott also knew disappointment. Among all the projects to improve nursing education and research, she never lost her vision of the influence of nursing to improve patient care. In the late 1960s, she developed an ambitious project to explore, design, and implement the extension of WCHEN activities beyond nursing education to nursing practice. Nearly 50 years ahead of her time, she prepared a proposal for funding to transform nursing practice. But the WICHE executive group declined to approve submission of the proposal, fearing that her vision was beyond the scope of the work of WICHE. Elliott noted this as the most significant "lost opportunity" of her 23 years at the organization (Abbott, 2004, p. 99 and note 22, p. 277). This and other many projects are well chronicled in other histories of the organization, and will not be explored in detail here (see WIN, 1992; 2007). The focus of this work is on the significant work of the organization to promote and communicate nursing research through its annual conference.

Annual Regional Conferences
As mentioned, Elliott immediately began yearly regional conferences on nursing issues. These came to be known as the WCHEN "annual conferences," and are not to be confused with the three regional conferences to be discussed below that were preliminary to the annual *Communicating Nursing Research* conference. They might be viewed as forerunners to what became the annual WIN Assembly conferences. The foresight and inclusiveness of the conferences are impressive. For example, participants included the presidents and other academic leaders of western universities; deans and chairs of nursing and other disciplines, such as medicine, sociology, anthropology, and political science; legislative personnel; hospital administrators; representatives from baccalaureate, associate degree, and diploma schools of nursing; representatives from national philanthropic organizations; and federal officials (see WCHEN, 1958; 1959; 1960; 1961).

The first conference was *Today, Tomorrow, The Day After That,* held in March 1958 in San Francisco. Attendance included 220 participants from 13 western states (WCHEN, 1958a). The second conference, *A Look Ahead for Western Nursing,* was held in April 1959 in Phoenix. Attendance was sustained at 225 participants.

Harold Enarson, Executive Director of WICHE, noted:

> The first purpose of this conference is to expose our thinking to people who think differently. We deliberately organized this conference today to attract not simply nursing educators, but consumers of nursing service as well. The second purpose is defined as suggesting specific next steps which the Western Interstate Commission for Higher Education, through the Nursing Council, should take here in the West (Enarson, 1959, p. 6).

The third conference, *Nurses for Tomorrow: Developing Actions Programs,* was held March 24-25, 1960 in Salt Lake City. Elliott noted that this conference "differed from its predecessors in having something new to talk to. This was the report *Nurses for the West,* the first study ever made of the nursing needs of a great region and of ways to meet these needs" (WCHEN, 1960, p. 3). Fourth and fifth conferences were held in Los Angeles and Boulder (WCHEN, 1961; 1962). These continued to include a large range of regional and national representatives from higher education, health care administration and practice, and funding sources. Though they were generally focused on nursing education issues, the importance of research to advance the profession was a continuing thread throughout the conferences. Elliott noted, "Special emphasis was given to research in nursing, which has a vital role to play in the improvement of nursing service" (Elliott, 1961, p. 2).

The Focus on Research: Seeds Planted for *Communicating Nursing Research*

From the beginning, the vision of an organization to advancing nursing in the West was comprehensive: to expand its focus on nursing education to include improvement to and access to programs, faculty development, continuing education, improvement of practice, and the development and dissemination of research. Early discussions always included a plan for some forum to advance and communicate nursing research.

Elliott secured funds from the United States Public Health Service to plan and conduct three regional conferences on research in nursing. The conferences were focused on development of researchers and their research: to promote research and explore methods to advance research, rather than to only report or critique actual research. Hoffman reported that the purpose of these conferences was to "expand nursing research" (Sorensen, 1992, p. 32) "through improvement of knowledge and skills of those who teach research methods and guide students in their skills" (Hoffman, 1968). The conferences included invited consultants from other disciplines, such as public health, biostatistics, social psychology, and sociology (Fry, 1958b; Sorensen, 1992).

The first conference was held at the University of Colorado for five days in December 1957 "for faculty who taught research methods and guided research" (WIN, 1992, p. 10). Participants included 27 faculty members representing the following institutions: College of Medical Evangelists, University of California Berkeley, University of California Los Angeles, University of Colorado, Montana State College, University of Washington, and University of Utah (Kelly, 1958, p. 3).

21

The following year, 1958, a second regional conference on research in nursing was held at the University of California Berkeley to "consider and plan for research projects in the area of patient care" (WIN, 1992, p. 10). Vera Fry reported that this conference reflected the forward thinking from the beginning to focus on patient care. Twenty nurses participated. "For two weeks these nurses worked arduously in small task-oriented groups on broad but appropriate models which might serve as the basis for definitive research designs" (Fry, 1958a; Fry, 1958c, p. 5).

Also in 1958, a third regional conference, *Ongoing Research Projects in Nursing in the Western Region,* was held at the University of Washington to exchange information on current research projects and to explore future projects (see WCHEN, 1958b). From this conference was created the *Report of Current Research in the Field of Nursing by Faculty of WCHEN Schools of Nursing* (WCHEN, 1963). McNeil and Lindeman (in press) noted that the report listed "66 ongoing studies, most of which (n=38, 57.6%) were directly related to patient care; 17 (25.8%) focused on nursing students, 10 (15.2%) on curriculum and teaching, and one on organization."

An important part of the 1958 conference in Washington was the report of Ellwynne Vreeland, Chief of Research Grants and Fellowships Branch of the Division of Nursing of the U. S. Public Health Service. She explained that since the beginning of the research grants program in 1955, a total of 54 research awards had been made to research related to nursing, though many of these were small seed grants of $2,300 or less. Perhaps more important at the time, 78 full-time nursing research fellowships had been granted. She added, "We can now do something about nursing problems we want solved and about young nurses with research promise" (Vreeland, 1958, pp. 178-179; See Note 1-D). As a result of this conference, documentation of current funded faculty research was completed and new research projects were begun (Elliott, 1992; Sorensen, 1992; WIN, 1992).

Elliott (1992, pp. 25-26) later explained, in her own words, WCHEN's focus on research from the "very beginning":

Fortuitously, in 1955 the federal government, through the United States Public Health Service (USPHS), initiated funding for nursing research. At the first meeting in March 1957 of the WCHEN Graduate Seminar (the dean plus one graduate faculty member from each graduate program, participation funded by the W. K. Kellogg Foundation grant) regional research efforts were begun. The seminar specified the research actions for the first priority. Responsibilities were assigned and/or assumed and grant applications were quickly submitted to the USPHS. Funding soon followed.

The University of Colorado carried out a project of three conferences (1957, 1959, 1961) designed to strengthen and expand effective research in nursing through improving the research knowledge and skills of the Western graduate faculty who were teaching research and/or guiding graduate students doing master's theses . . .

The second effort was a two week workshop/conference conducted in January 1958 by the School of Public Health, University of California, Berkeley, plus the Schools of Nursing at UCSF and UCLA. Twenty nurses from service and education participated. They represented ten university schools of nursing, two state health departments, three city health departments, one Veterans Administration hospital, and the Army Nurse Corps. . .

The University of Washington carried out the third regional effort, a conference held in late April 1958: *Ongoing Research Projects in Nursing in the Western Region.* Individual ongoing studies were reported; consultants from psychology, sociology, and education commented on and appraised the work (One psychologist told the group there would <u>never</u> be a science of nursing! He said that nurses should identify the problems and let psychology and sociology study them. By the third Colorado conference, 1961, he revised his words to say that there are some questions so unique to patient care and nursing that only nurses can study them!). Of all the regional work in research prior to 1968, the University of Washington conference is most nearly the forerunner of the annual regional research conferences . . .

Leininger (1992, p. 45) later confirmed the early challenges to establishing a recognized science of nursing:

. . . [S]ome of the biggest skeptics were non-nurse researchers from other disciplines who had never entered the world of nursing and who had great difficulty envisioning nursing phenomena and ways that nurses could do research without a "legitimate scientist" with them. I well remember a sociologist who constantly reminded me that nurses must be fully socialized about the methods used by "legitimate scientists" in order for their work to be accepted or recognized. While these colleagues from other disciplines have been enormously helpful to demonstrate scientific research, they also seemed to want to keep nurses figuratively "under their wings" in order to monitor and protect them. But it was time for nurses "to fly it alone."

Hoffman (1968, p. 16) confirmed the resistance and lamented that one of the consultants presumptuously announced:

There is a profession of nursing, but there is not now or never will be a science of nursing. Nursing contributes to the formation of the research problem, nurses participate in liaison with the research worker; but studies are carried out by research workers competent in the field in which the research problem lies.

Following are the very words from one consultant to the conference, Kenneth Hammond, Associate Professor of Psychology at the University of Colorado and Visiting Associate Professor of Psychology at the University of California Berkeley:

As I listened to the research reports yesterday I developed a certain sense of uneasiness about what is called "nursing research," or "research in nursing." After thinking about this matter following yesterday's conference, the reason for my uneasiness has become apparent to me . . .

I believe that those individuals who are guiding the profession of nursing into the field of research are making a serious mistake . . .

23

Instead of leaving the actual execution of the research to those trained in the particular field in which the problems lies, nurses are being urged to "do-it-yourself" . . . There is a profession of nursing, but there is not now and never will be a science of nursing . . .

If they wish to do research in chemistry—let them become chemists, with a Ph.D. in chemistry, not nursing. If they wish to do research in education, let them earn a Ph.D. in education, not nursing . . . What can a Ph.D. in nursing possibly mean? (WCHEN, 1960, pp. 77-79).

In spite of such resistance, Elliott and WCHEN persisted:

The Western Council on Higher Education for Nursing is a demonstration that schools can work together. One aspect of interschool cooperation is sharing knowledge of the ongoing research and problems encountered in conduction research in other parts of the region . . . [S]tudy and research cannot be separate from each other in schools of nursing if the West is to contribute to the body of knowledge of nursing through research activities . . . Regional research conferences emphasize the growing responsibility that schools of nursing have for initiating and conducting research . . .

A regional conference provides opportunity for faculty members directly involved in research . . . to share the stimulation and current progress of others in similar institutions . . .

[W]hat is even more important . . . has been the willingness of people to "expose" themselves and their research problems to the criticism of their peers and consultants. This may reflect the spirit of the West, as well as regional cooperation—trying the new and untried, seeking constructive criticism, accepting setbacks or failure as only temporary blocks to progress, but striving toward improvement with enthusiasm and interest (WCHEN, 1960, pp. 174-175).

It is worth inserting, and now obvious, that from the beginning, early Keynote presentations of the *Communicating Nursing Research* conference soon debunked such perspectives (see Appendix A). And on into the future, the Keynote, Distinguished Research Lectureships, New Researcher presentations, thousands of high-level research presentations at the conference (see Appendices), and the stature of its offspring, the *Western Journal of Nursing Research,* further nullified such notions that nursing may not be a science.

Second Executive Director of WICHE: Robert Kroepsch

In 1960, Enarson retired from leadership of WICHE. He had established a strong and stable organization, leaving all 13 states as members and staff in place. Robert Kroepsch came to WICHE in 1960 as the second Executive Director. His roots were on the east coast, having served the previous for five years with the New England Board of Higher Education. He was accustomed to working with the old, private, and prestigious colleges and universities of the East, having himself graduated from Bates College, a small, highly-ranked, liberal arts school in Lewiston, Maine (Kroepsch Award, 2016). He found that "in the West on the other hand, it was the public universities that were dominant in esteem" (Abbott, 2004, p. 77). Nevertheless, he brought his Associate Director, Kevin Bunnell, to "engage in an experiment" (Abbott, 2004, p. 77), and reported to the Commissioners that he was "delighted with the spirit" he found at WICHE (Abbott, 2004, p. 78).

Kroepsch led WICHE for 16 years, until 1976. He announced his retirement rather suddenly at the unfortunate news of the cancer diagnosis of his beloved wife, Ruth. She died in 1975. In 1985, honoring his wife, he established the Kroepsch Award for Excellence in Teaching at his alma mater, Bates College (Kroepsch Award, 2016). In 1971, the College awarded him the honorary doctor of laws (LL.D) degree (Bates College, 1971). He was known for frugality and as a popular commencement speaker throughout the United States (Burns, 2013, p. 9). He died in 1986.

Abbott (2004, p. 239) confirmed, "The Nursing Program was a Kroepsch favorite. Its director, Jo Eleanor Elliott was full of ideas and of energy, and the program was continually moving into issues that lay at the heart of nursing education and that called attention to WICHE." Kroepsch continued to support nursing and WCHEN projects. He admired the energy of Jo Eleanor Elliott as a "go-getter" (Abbott, 2004, p. 78), and benefited from her regional and national influence. For example, in 1962 Kroepsch was invited to address 1,500 attendees at the convention of the National Student Nurses Association; and Kevin Bunnell gave the Keynote speech at the National Health Careers Conference. In 1964, Kroepsch received a letter from the W. K. Kellogg Foundation stating, "WICHE appears to be the greatest dynamic force for nursing in this country at the present time" (Abbott, 2004, p. 96). In 1966, Kroepsch changed Elliott's title from "nurse consultant" to "director of nursing programs," an action seen as "long overdue" and likely an indicator of the continuing gender inequality in higher education at the time (Abbott, 2004, p. 96).

The Vision of *Communicating Nursing Research* Becomes a Reality
By 1961, The W. K. Kellogg Foundation provided support for five additional years (WIN, 1992, p. 11). At the end of the five years when funding ended, the WICHE Commission agreed to support the continuation of the Nursing Program.

Progress continued over the next eight years with projects related to baccalaureate program content, a survey of nursing needs, a leadership program, and other specific research-based projects. Among them was a 12-year annual report, *Current Research in WCHEN Schools*, that led to the report *Newly Initiated and Completed Research by Faculty of WCHEN Schools of Nursing* as efforts to promote networking of emerging nurse researchers in the West (Elliott, 1992). Also, Elliott led an annual *Western Conference on Nursing Education* that was highly inclusive of health professionals in the region. In addition, in 1965, Elliott was recruited by colleges of the Mid-Atlantic States for guidance to create a "WCHEN-like structure" (Abbott, 2004, p. 96). Always with an eye toward an annual conference focused on research, funding was secured to make the vision a continuing reality. By 1968, federal funds were obtained to provide three annual conferences. The success of the first three sessions laid the foundation for a competitive renewal of funding for an additional three annual conferences. Thus, the annual *Communicating Nursing Research* conference was born.

References

Abbott, F. C. (2004). *A history of the Western Interstate Commission for Higher Education: The first 40 years.* Boulder, CO: WICHE. See Note 1-D.

Abdellah, F. G., Beland, I. I., Martin, A., & Matheney, R. V. (1960). *Patient-centered approaches in nursing.* New York City, NY: Macmillan.

Abdellah, F. G., & Levine, E. (1965). Better patient care through nursing research. *International Journal of Nursing Studies, 2,* 1-12.

American Nurses Association (ANA). (1984). Elwynne Mae Vreeland (1909-1971), 194 Inductee. *ANA Hall of fame inductees.* Retrieved February 1, 2017 from www.nursingworld.org/EllwynneMaeVreeland.

American Nurses Association (ANA). (2012). RADM Faye Glenn Abdellah, (Ret.) USPHS, EdD, ScD, RN, FAAN, 2012 inductee. *American Nurses Association Hall of Fame inductees.* Retrieved August 23, 2016 from http://www.nursingworld. org/fayeglennabdellah.

American Nurses Association (ANA). (2016). Katherine J. Hoffman (1910-1984), 1996 inductee. *American Nurses Association Hall of Fame inductees.* Retrieved August 17, 2016 from http://www.nursingworld.org/KatherineJHoffman.

Anderson, H. (1975, May 22-28). Enochs retires to Oregon. *Sonoma State Morning Glory, 11(17),* 1. Courtesy of Sonoma State University Archives.

Anderson, N. (2015, April). Hanna Basin Museum honors Amelia Leino and Lillian Turner. *Hanna Basin Museum.* Retrieved August 17, 2016 from http://www. hannabasinmuseum.com/-amelia-leino-and-lillian-truner-exhibit.html.

Associated Press. (2006, August 1). Sports: Harold Enarson, 87, who fired Woody Hayes at Ohio State, dies. *New York Times*, B7. Retrieved August 16, 2016 from http://www.nytimes.com/2006/08/01/sports/01enarson.html?_r=0.

Bak, G. P. (2011, June). Jo Eleanor Elliott: A legacy of courage. *American Nurse Today, 6(6).*

Bates College. (1971, June 1). *List of Honorary Degree Recipients.* Retrieved January 11, 2017 from http://www.bates.edu/president/list-of-honorary-degree-recipients/.

Burns, H. J. (2013, March 10). Bates in brief college: The man behind the Kroepsch name. *Bates Magazine.* Lewiston, ME: Bates College. Retrieved January 16, 2017 from http://www.bates.edu/news/2013/03/10/bates-in-brief-college-the-man-behind-the-kroepsch-name/.

Cipriano, P. F. (2011, June). Editorial. *American Nurse Today, 6(6).*

College of Health & Human Sciences. (2007). *Northern Illinois University School of Nursing Annette Lefkowitz fund for nursing research.* Retrieved from www.chhs. niu.edu/nursing/_documents/Lefkowitz07.pdf.

Coulter, P. P. (1963, July). *The winds of change: Progress report of regional cooperation in collegiate nursing education in the West.* Boulder, CO: WICHE. WIN archives, Portland, OR.

Culver, V. (2011, May 3). Health care, nursing activist Jo Elliott won Obama's praise. *Denver Post.* Retrieved August 23, 2016 from http://www.denverpost. com/2011/05/03/health-care-nursing-activist-jo-elliott-won-obamas-praise/.

Curtin, L. (2011, July 12). One thought on "Jo Eleanor Elliott: A legacy of courage." *American Nurse Today, 6(6).*

Denogean, A. T. (2002, February 7). Obituary: Pearl Coulter, first dean of UA College of Nursing. *Tucson Citizen* (archive). Retrieved August 17, 2016 from http:// tucsoncitizen.com/morgue2/2002/02/07/179481-obituary/.

Denver Post. (2011, May 4). Obituary: Jo Eleanor Elliott. Retrieved August 23, 2016 from http://www.legacy.com/obituaries/denverpost/obituary.aspx?pid+150772184.

Dunphy, L. (2009). "With the very best of intentions:" The development of nursing process as a way of knowing. In R. C. Locsin & M. J. Purnell, *A contemporary nursing process: The (un)bearable weight of knowing in nursing* (pp. 31-60). New York City, NY: Springer.

Elliott, J. E. (1959). *Nurses for the West.* Boulder, CO: WICHE & WCHEN.

Elliott, J. E. (1961). Foreword. In *Fourth annual western conference on nursing education: Dilemmas in nursing.* Los Angeles, CA. Proceedings (p. 2). WIN Archives: Portland, OR.

Elliott, J. E. (1966, July). The profession prepares for the future. *American Journal of Nursing, 66(7),* 1548-1567.

Elliott, J. E. (1992). The West's regional efforts in nursing research. In *The anniversary book: A history of nursing in the West 1956-1992* (pp. 25-30). Boulder, CO: WIN.

Enarson, H. L. (1959, April 16). *Nursing in the West: Facts and figures.* Address at regional WCHEN conference. WIN Archives: Portland, OR.

Find a grave memorial. (2010). Harold L. Enarson # 56903108. Retrieved July 14, 2016 from http://www.findagrave.com/cgi-bin/fg.cgi?page=gr&Grid=56903108.

Fry, V. (1953). A creative approach to nursing. *American Journal of Nursing, 53, 3,* 301-302.

Fry, V. (1958a, January 20-February 1). Conference on research in nursing. WIN Archives, Portland, OR.

Fry, V. (1958b). *Conference on research in nursing proceedings.* Boulder, CO: WICHE. WIN Archives, Portland, OR.

Fry, V. (1958c). Report of second regional conference. In *Ongoing research projects in nursing in the western region,* Seattle, WA. Proceedings (pp. 5-6). Boulder, CO: WCHEN. WIN Archives, Portland, OR.

Hoffman, K. J. (1968). Changing approaches to nursing research in the West. In M. V. Batey (Ed.), *Communicating Nursing Research, 1* (pp. 13-19). Boulder, CO: WCHEN.

Humphrey, G. (2002, February 6). Nursing education pioneer Pearl Parvin Coulter, founding dean of UA College of Nursing, dies at 99. *Office of Public Affairs, University of Arizona.* Retrieved August 16, 2016 from http://opa.ahsc.arizona. edu/newsroom/news/2002/nursing-education-pioneer-pearl-parvin-coulter-founding-dean-ua-college-nursing-d.

James Enochs Papers. (1999). *Guide to the James Enochs papers.* Online Archive of California, California State University, Dominguez Hills Archives. Retrieved January 29, 2017 from http://www.oac.cdlib.org/findaid/ark:/13030/tf996nb384/entire_text/.

Jersey Shore University Medical Center (2016). *Our history.* Retrieved August 23, 2016 from http://www.jerseyshoreuniversitymedicalcenter.com/jsumc/aboutus/ourhistory.cfm.

Jo Eleanor Elliott is named to national post. (1980, September-October). *Sigma Theta Tau Reflections, 6,* 1. Retrieved August 23, 2016 from http://www.nursinglibrary.org/vhl/handle/10755/560920.

Kelly, K. (1958). Report of first regional conference. In *Ongoing research projects in nursing in the western region,* Seattle, WA. Proceedings (pp. 3-4). Boulder, CO: WCHEN. WIN Archives, Portland, OR.

Kroepsch Award (2016). *Dean of the faculty.* Retrieved January 11, 2017 from https://www.bates.edu/dof/news-and-calendars/kroepsch-award/.

Leininger, M. (1992). Reflections on WCHEN and *The Research Critique.* In *The anniversary book: A history of nursing in the West 1956-1992* (pp. 43-49). Boulder, CO: WIN.

Marsh, J. T. (1969). Nursing school celebrates 10 years of progress. *Northern Illinois University News Items, 20(10),* 4.

McConnell, T. R., Holy, T. C., & Semans, H. H. (1955). *A restudy of the needs of California in higher education.* University Archives, The Bancroft Library, University of California at Berkeley. Retrieved January 29, 2017 from http://content. cdlib.org/view?docld=hb2n39n7ns&chunk.id=tpage&brand=calisphere&doc. view=entire_text.

McNeil, P. A., & Lindeman, C. A. (in press). A history of the Western Institute of Nursing and its *Communicating Nursing Research* conferences. *Nursing Research.*

Mirsky, Z., Olesen, V., & Weiss, S. J. (1992). Helen Nahm, nursing: San Francisco. In D. Krogh (Ed.), *University of California: In memoriam, 1992.* Retrieved August 16, 2016 from http://texts.cdlib.org/view?docid=hb7c6007sj;NAAN=13030& doc.view=frames&chunk.id=div00046&tox.depth=1&toc.id=brand=calisphere.

Nahm, H. (1956). The problem: Improvement in nursing services and education in the West: A report of visits to colleges and universities in the Western area. Reprinted as Appendix A from *Toward shared planning in Western nursing education,* WICHE in P. P. Coulter *The winds of change* (pp. 47-58). Boulder, CO: WICHE. WIN archives, Portland, OR.

Napa Valley Register. (2004, March 20). Obituaries: Kathryn Lastreto. Retrieved August 17, 2016 from http://napavalleyregister.com/news/local/obituaries/ kathryn-lastreto/article_f7c30b13-8574-5961-aa7b-02e7479dde5c.html.

National League for Nursing (NLN Report). (1971, November). *NLN Department of Baccalaureate and Higher Degree Programs record of nurse faculty and instructional staff member.* Northern Illinois University School of Nursing Archives.

National Women's Hall of Fame. (2016). *Faye Glenn Abdellah.* Seneca Falls, NY: National Women's Hall of Fame. Retrieved August 23, 2016 from https://www. womenofthehall.org/inductee/faye-glenn-abdellah/.

New York University (NYU) College of Nursing. (2016). Retrieved August 16, 2016 from http://ec2-184-73-211-184.compute-1.amazonaws.com/index.php/New_ York_University_College_of_Nursing.

New York University (NYU) Rory Meyers College of Nursing. (2016). Retrieved August 16, 2016 from https://en/wikipedia.org/wiki/New_York_University_ Rory_Meyers_College_of_Nursing.

News-Press. (2001, July 15). Death notice: Annette Lefkowitz. Retrieved January 16, 2017 from http://www.legacy.com/obituaries/news-press/obituary. aspx?n=annette-lefkowitz&pid=18631649.

Northern Illinois School of Nursing celebrates 50 years. (2009, October 14-20). *The Rock River Times.* Retrieved January 16, 2017 from http://rockrivertimes. com/wpapp/online-exclusives/2009/10/14/northern-illinois-school-of-nursing-celebrates-50-years/.

Oliver, M. (1995, September 1). Obituaries: Lulu Hassenplug; Founded UCLA School of Nursing. *Los Angeles Times.*

Online archive of California. (2016). Register of the Helen Nahm Papers, 1922-1977. Retrieved August 16, 2016 from http://www.oac.cdlib.org/findaid/ark:/13030/ tf709nb51w/.

Pair, Nona T. (1966, April). *Today and tomorrow in Western nursing.* Boulder, CO: WICHE.

Sachs, A. (2011, May 3). ANA mourns past president Jo Eleanor Elliott. *News Release.* Silver Spring, MD: American Nurses Association. Retrieved August 23, 2016 from http://www.nursingworld.org/FunctionalMenuCategories/MediaResources/PressReleases/2011-PR/ANA-Mourns-Jo-Eleanor-Elliott.pdf.

Schwartz, A. (2014, July). Profiles in nursing: Seeking Helen Nahm: Visionary established nursing as its own unique discipline. *Science of caring: A publication of the UCSF School of Nursing.* Retrieved August 16, 2016 from http://scienceofcaring.ucsf.edu/profiles-nursing/seeking-helen-nahm-visionary-established-nursing-its-own-unique=-discipline.

Shipley, S. (1980). Lulu Hassenplug. In *VUMC through time.* Retrieved May 18, 2016 from https://www.mc.vanderbilt.edu/throughtime/items/show/11770.

Smith, K. M. (1956, March 30). Letter to H. Enarson. WIN Archives, Portland, OR.

Sonoma State University (SSU). (2016). History of SSU. Retrieved February 1, 2017 from www.sonoma.edu/about/history/html.

Sorensen, G. E. (1992). Faculty development in nursing research: Historical overview. In *The anniversary book: A history of nursing in the west 1956-1992* (pp. 31-36). Boulder, CO: WIN.

University of Arizona. (2002, April 18). Memorial service for nursing education pioneer Pearl Parvin Coulter, April 25. *UA News.* Retrieved August 16, 2016 from https://uanews.arizona.edu/story/memorial-service-nursing-eduation=-pioneer-pearl-parvin-coulter-april-25.

University of California San Francisco (UCSF). (2016). People: Helen Nahm. (2016). *A History of UCSF.* Retrieved August 16, 2016 from http://history.library.ucsf.edu/nahm.html.

University of Colorado at Denver (CU). (2005, January). In memoriam: Kathryn Smith Lastreto, SON dean 1965-1974. *University of Colorado at Denver & Health Sciences Center School of Nursing News, 5.*

University of Wyoming. (2001). *History of the University of Wyoming School of Nursing.* Retrieved August 17, 2016 from http://www.uwyo.edu/nursing/about-our-school-history.html.

Vreeland, E. (1958). Comments on conference. *Ongoing research projects in nursing in the western region,* Seattle, WA. Proceedings (pp. 176-179). Boulder, CO: WCHEN. WIN Archives, Portland, OR

Washington State Nurses Association (WSNA). (1996). Katherine J. Hoffman. *WSNA hall of fame.* Retrieved August 17, 2016 from https://www.wsna.org/hall-of-fame/1996/Katherine-Hoffman/.

Washington State Nurses Association (WSNA). (2004). Marjorie Batey. *WSNA hall of fame.* Retrieved August 17, 2016 from https://www.wsna.org/hall-of-fame/2004/marjorie-batey.

Western Council on Higher Education for Nursing (WCHEN) (1957). *Charter of the Western Council on Higher Education for Nursing of the Western Interstate Commission for Higher Education.* Boulder, CO: WICHE. In P. P. Coulter (1963, July), *The winds of change* (Appendix C, pp. 63-66). Boulder, CO: WICHE. WIN archives, Portland, OR. Also in WIN (2007). *The anniversary book: 50 years of advancing nursing in the West 1957-2007* (pp. 27-36). Portland, OR: WIN.

Western Council on Higher Education for Nursing (WCHEN). (1958a, March 16-17). *Nursing education: Today, tomorrow, the day after that,* San Francisco, CA. Proceedings. WIN Archives: Portland, OR.

Western Council on Higher Education for Nursing (WCHEN). (1958b, April 30-May 2). *Ongoing research projects in nursing in the western region,* Seattle, WA. Proceedings. WIN Archives, Portland, OR.

Western Council on Higher Education for Nursing (WCHEN). (1959, April 16-17). *Second annual western conference on nursing education: A look ahead for Western nursing*, Phoenix, AZ. Program. WIN Archives: Portland, OR.

Western Council on Higher Education for Nursing (WCHEN). (1960, March 24-25). *Third annual western conference on nursing education: Nurses for tomorrow: Developing action programs*, Salt Lake City, UT. WIN Archives: Portland, OR.

Western Council on Higher Education for Nursing (WCHEN). (1961, March 9-10). *Fourth annual western conference on nursing education: Dilemmas in nursing.* Los Angeles, CA. Proceedings. WIN Archives: Portland, OR.

Western Council on Higher Education for Nursing (WCHEN). (1962, March 22-23). *Fifth annual western conference on nursing education: The pursuit of excellence in nursing.* Boulder, CO. Proceedings. WIN Archives, Portland, OR.

Western Council on Higher Education for Nursing (WCHEN). (1963). *Report of current research in the field of nursing by faculty of WCHEN schools of nursing.* WIN Archives, Portland, OR.

Western Institute of Nursing (WIN). (1992). *The anniversary book: A history of nursing in the West: 1956-1992.* Boulder, CO: WIN.

Western Institute of Nursing (WIN). (2007). *The anniversary book: 50 years of advancing nursing in the west 1957-2007.* Portland, OR: WIN.

Western Institute of Nursing (WIN). (2016a). About WIN: History of WIN. Retrieved January 22, 2017 from https://www.winursing.org/about-win/.

Western Institute of Nursing (WIN). (2016b). History subcommittee: Potential interviewees for the 50th anniversary project. WIN Archives, Portland, OR.

Western Institute of Nursing (WIN). (2016c). *Jo Eleanor Elliott leadership award.* Retrieved August 23, 2016 from http://winursing.org/?query=jeela.

Western Institute of Nursing (WIN). (2016c). *WIN Emeriti.* Retrieved August 17, 2016 from http://winursing.org/?query=WIN+Emeriti.

Western Interstate Commission for Higher Education (WICHE). (1961, March 9-10). *Fourth annual Western Conference on Nursing Education: Dilemmas in nursing,* Los Angeles, CA. WIN Archives, Portland, OR.

Western Interstate Commission for Higher Education (WICHE). (1969, January). *Annual report: 1968.* Boulder, CO: WICHE. Retrieved August 17, 2016 from http://files.eric.ed.gov/fulltext/ED027013.pdf.

Western Interstate Commission for Higher Education (WICHE). (2016). *About WICHE.* Boulder, CO: WICHE. Retrieved July 14, 2016 from http://www.wiche.edu/about.

Notes

1-A. The original 13 state members of WICHE were the following, in alphabetical order: Alaska, Arizona, California, Colorado, Hawaii, Idaho, Montana, Nevada, New Mexico, Oregon, Utah, Washington, and Wyoming.

1-B. Current membership in WICHE includes the following: Alaska, Arizona, California, Colorado, Hawaii, Idaho, Montana, Nevada, New Mexico, North Dakota, Oregon, South Dakota, Utah, Washington, and Wyoming (see WICHE, 2015. Retrieved August 16, 2016 from http://www.wiche.edu/forum/membership/current) and the Northern Mariana Islands (see WICHE, 2015b. Retrieved August 16, 2016 from http://www.wiche.edu/wiche-region/cnmi).

1-C. Coulter (1963, p. 24) noted that a revision of the WCHEN charter in March, 1962 "provided for an Associate Degree Seminar." The Western Institute of Nursing (WIN) has since expanded to invite representatives from all nursing education programs in the region as well as clinical agencies.

1-D. Ellwynne Vreeland, Chief, Research Grants Branch, Division of Nursing Resources, Department of Health, Education, and Welfare, United States Public Health Service, called this conference "the first one of its kind conducted in the field of nursing" (see Fry, 1958a). Vreeland went on to be instrumental in the development and implementation of the first nationwide federal extramural research program for nursing and was an early proponent of the National Institute of Nursing Research (see ANA, 1984).

1-E. Abbott's *A history of the Western Interstate Commission for Higher Education: The first 40 years,* has no date of publication indicated anywhere within the volume. Several informal sources (contemporaries who have signed, dates copies; calculations of events covered; and general consensus among contemporaries) confirm that the publication date should be 2004, and thus is listed as such.

Chapter Two

LAUNCHING *Communicating Nursing Research*, 1968-1973

Chapter Two
LAUNCHING *Communicating Nursing Research,* 1968-1973

To launch an annual research conference was the culmination of just one of the significant plans and dreams to improve health care and advance nursing in the West. Western leaders were pioneers, projecting amazing foresight to begin the *Communicating Nursing Research* series, the first of its kind in the United States (WIN, 2016a). Juanita Murphy noted that "nurse researchers in the West are viewed by colleagues across the nation as the forerunners of the second phase of scientific nursing" (Murphy, 1992, p. 37).

There were few national models for successful conferences to disseminate nursing research. Nursing research itself was in its infancy. In 1965, the American Nurses Association had begun federally funded research conferences (Editorial, 1965), but questions about their quality and/or effectiveness provoked continued interest in a conference in the West (see Benoliel, 1992, p. 126; Elliott, 1992, p. 28).

The early leaders were thoughtful in planning a conference series not only for the present, but for the future. They began with attention to research development and promotion of doctoral education among nurse educators in the West. Besides the foundation in research development among its members, other unique strengths at the outset of the conference have continued through its history. The inclusion of critique of presentations in the very first session was remarkable and viewed as "peer evaluation of research as a necessary component of the research process" (Murphy, 1992, p. 39). The concept eventually contributed to the format for one of the first research-focused academic journals, *Western Journal for Nursing Research* (see Brink, 1992). Also, the compilation of a professional conference proceedings that eventually became an important annual publication was significant.

The conference was envisioned and executed by people. It is the people who make the story: leaders in nursing who were collaborative and at the same time competitive, all trying to improve health and advance nursing as a profession by building and sharing its science.

Jeanne Quint Benoliel confirmed (1992, p. 125):

Trying to capture in language the climate of any coming together of people in a conference is hard to do because the nuances of feelings, the dynamics of interpersonal transactions, and the underlying power games among those seeking prestige and control do not translate easily into written work (except perhaps in novels). People dynamics at the . . . conferences always have been fascinating and, in fact, have contributed to the vitality of these annual meetings.

And Marjorie Batey (1992, p. 54) noted:

The richness of the conferences has been through the interchange of ideas, the formation of colleagueships among persons of like and of different conceptual and methodological interests . . . and the mentoring that has occurred between persons of different experience backgrounds.

The Visionaries and Visionary Planning

With federal funding from the Division of Nursing secured by Jo Eleanor Elliott, a planning committee was appointed to begin the work. Mildred Quinn, from Utah, served as Chair of the Western Council on Higher Education for Nursing (WCHEN) Executive Committee (1967-1968). The Conference Planning Committee included Katherine Hoffman (an original member of the first Committee of Seven described in Chapter 1), Madeleine Leininger, and R. Maureen Maxwell, with Marjorie Batey as WCHEN Project Director (WIN, 1992, p. 393).

Mildred D. R. Quinn was a citizen of the West. She was born in Liberty, Idaho and graduated from Salt Lake County Hospital School of Nursing in 1922 and the University of Oregon in 1942. She earned the M.S. at the University of Utah in 1946 and a doctorate from Teachers College at Columbia University in 1952. She was the first instructor appointed to the Department of Nursing in the School of Education at the University of Utah (Clayton, 2000). She was the second dean of the College of Nursing at the University of Utah, where she served from 1954 to 1973. Under her leadership, the College established the M.S. degree and clinical sites among Navajo communities for training of nurse midwives and pediatric nurses. She was active as a professional author and editor and most proud of her work on the College of Nursing building that stands today. She was the only person to serve two separate terms as Chair of WCHEN/WIN (1959-1960 and 1967-1968) (WIN, 2016c). She died in 2000 in Utah at the age of 92 (Deseret News, 2000).

Madeleine Leininger was born on a farm near Sutton, Nebraska, joined the United States Army Nursing Corps, and graduated from St. Anthony's School of Nursing in Denver, Colorado. She earned the B.S. from St. Scholastica Benedictine College in Atchison, Kansas, M.S. from Catholic University in Washington DC, and the Ph.D. in cultural and social anthropology from the University of Washington (Johnson, 2012). She was eventually the visionary and "foundress" of the Transcultural Nursing Society, well-known nursing theorist, and prolific author. She was professor at Wayne State University, dean of the schools of nursing at the University of Washington and the University of Utah, President of the American Association of Colleges of Nursing, and finally returned to her home as professor at the University of Nebraska before her death in 2012 (see Johnson, 2012; UNMC, 2012; Nurse.com, 2012).

R. Maureen Maxwell was a beloved faculty member at Loma Linda University in California, where today a student scholarship bears her name. Her writings focused on nursing education and preparation of faculty. The year of the first conference, she published on preparation of teachers of nursing (see Maxwell, 1968b). She was described as a "warm, personable individual" and "a solid, contributing member of the conference committee" through its first five years (M. V. Batey, personal communication, September 10, 2016). She was elected Chair of WCHEN 1965-1966 (WIN, 2016c).

Marjorie Batey was born in Hamburg, Iowa, raised in Nebraska, and graduated from Sacred Heart Hospital School of Nursing in Spokane, Washington. She earned the B.S. in nursing from the University of Washington, M.S. in psychiatric nursing and the Ph.D. in sociology from the University of Colorado in Boulder. As Project Director for Nursing Research Programs for WICHE, she served on the Conference Planning Committee for its first six years and edited the first ten volumes of *Communicating*

Nursing Research, an experience that she once referred to as her "ten lost summers" (Batey, 1992, p. 51; Batey, September 10, 2016, personal communication). To this work she brought the experience of faculty member at the University of Colorado School of Nursing and at the University of Washington. She was among the first nurses in the west to earn the Ph.D. and among the pioneers to secure federal funding for research development, which she used to establish the organizational conditions essential to a strong environment for faculty research (WSNA, 2004).

Remembering the foundational work for the conference, Batey (1992, pp. 51-52) described:

> This conference series did not just happen. Rather, its beginning in 1968 can be seen as the culmination of a dynamic interaction of events and personalities that had been shaping higher education in nursing in the West throughout the 1950s and 1960s. Within that interaction, higher education in nursing and nursing research consistently were interwoven through their mutually supportive aims.

> We were fortunate in those early years to have nursing leaders with vision and who knew an opportunity when it came their way. . . With the formation of WCHEN, the Graduate Seminar within it, there was a structure for drawing together the deans, directors, and faculty of graduate programs in nursing to work on shared concerns and problems. The specific purposes of that structure were "the improvement of the quality of nursing research in the West and the improvement of the preparation of those who teach and/or conduct nursing research" (Elliott, 1968).

> But a structure alone could not accomplish the challenge that WCHEN had set for itself. Financial resources also were essential. While baseline support came through dues from member schools of nursing, it was not sufficient to develop faculty and to create and implement regional programs consistent with WCHEN's research purposes. How opportune it was that what was to become the Division of Nursing within the U. S. Public Health Service also was evolving in the early 1950s. The overlap of research program goals between WCHEN and the Division of Nursing was remarkable.

Benoliel (1992, p. 125) reported that participation in the first conferences was mostly "invitational and attendance ranged from 61 in 1968 to 103 in 1973." Benoliel (1992, p. 126) further recalled:

> To my recollection, the atmosphere of the early conferences was somewhat tense, probably because the presenters and critics had limited experience . . . Some of the critiques were constructive and focused; others were picky and harsh . . . Overall, the early conferences conveyed a sense of self-consciousness that, to my mind, was tied to the newness of the activity for many participants. At the same time there was much opportunity for people from many parts of the Western region to get acquainted and to lay the groundwork for future research and practice networks. These conferences provided a meeting place for a new generation of nurses who would become leaders in the future with the people who had paved the way.

More Than Just "Proceedings:" 50 Volumes of *Communicating Nursing Research*
Among the most visionary actions of the WCHEN pioneers was the decision to publish a first-class annual conference volume and engage a devoted editor from the beginning. Unlike most conference proceedings, even today, the nearly 50 volumes continue to be valuable resources for researchers for topics, methods, and collegial contacts. They include Keynote Addresses, New Researcher Award papers, Distinguished Research Lectures and State of the Science presentations that have become classics in the research literature of the discipline. They document the wisdom of seasoned scholars and the innovation of novice researchers. They provide a view of patterns, evolution, and growth of the science of nursing; and they continue to provide a treasure of historical archives on the progress of the discipline. Indeed, much of this very history is derived from the reports and first-hand accounts from the last 50 years of conference proceedings and associated "Anniversary Books" of the 25th and 50th anniversaries of WCHEN/WIN.

The first ten volumes of *Communicating Nursing Research* were compiled and edited by Marjorie Batey. She reflected:

> There are two primary purposes of the conference proceedings: 1) to document what occurred and 2) to extend the audience of the subject matter of the conference beyond those who attended . . . I believe both purposes were fulfilled . . . [R]eview of citations of published nursing studies reveals that there was extensive use of the papers from these conferences. Also, it is my impression that the proceedings have been used extensively as teaching references in graduate courses (Batey, 1992, p. 54).

The value of the volumes has exceeded Batey's vision. They are found on the shelves of the offices of nurse researchers throughout the country and in the best academic libraries. They continue to provide a rich resource to trace the patterns of the history of issues and research in the discipline of nursing.

The First Conference, 1968: *The Research Critique* – Salt Lake City, Utah

The vision of the conference series was to "communicate" nursing research. But a chasm lurked between organizational and professional values and vision and the reality of the dearth of advanced preparation of faculty to design, conduct, disseminate and produce a rich body of completed research for application to improve patient care. There was much work to be done to develop productive researchers. Elliott (1990, p. 3) reported that in 1968 about 500 nurses in the entire country held doctorates, and only 50 of those were in the West. Batey (1992, p. 53) explained:

> . . . [T]here was still a significant gap between what we would do, i.e. communicate findings of completed studies, and our espoused value, i.e. improving nursing practice. This set of conferences . . . would emphasize the research, not the development of persons. However, the Planning Committee . . . devised a plan through which the development of persons and a community of scholars would be a covert thrust of each conference.

> The foundation was laid with the first conference focusing on the research critique . . . Madeleine Leininger was charged with the Keynote Address that was to set the learning theme for the conference. Findings alone

were not the concern. Rather interest was in the credibility of the findings relative to all aspects of the study presented. Studies were to be presented, but they were to be examined carefully and constructively for the credibility of the findings both by a designated critic and by the participants . . . [The] intention was for the environment of the conferences to convey constructiveness and colleagueship.

The structure and execution of the conference reflected the consistent mission and themes of the original charter of WCHEN. Benoliel (1992, p. 125) observed:

The first six conferences came into being out of the thinking of nurse leaders in the WCHEN Graduate Seminar. These leaders were working very hard to establish nursing's credentials for membership in the academic community, and the push for nurses to do research was part of that effort. The conferences came from the efforts of people . . . called visionary nurses.

The conference began with an introduction to the current state of research in higher education by Kevin Bunnell, WICHE Associate Director and Director of Medical Education Programs. Katherine Hoffman then reported on the preliminary conferences leading to this series: "The Boulder Conferences," the "Berkley Conference," and the "Seattle Conference" (Batey, 1968a).

Batey (personal communication, February 17, 2016) further reflected:

The first session of [the] *Communicating Nursing Research Conference* series was called to order by Jo Eleanor Elliott on May 1, 1968 in Salt Lake City, Utah (Batey, 1968b, p. v) . . .

The format for the conference was so different from today's standards, but it reflected where we were in our early days of developing nursing research. The call for abstracts resulted in submissions from which five studies were selected for presentation. Each study was to be followed by a critique. Drawing from experiences of previous conferences that members of the planning committee had attended, it was decided that THIS conference series was to have a positive tone. It was to be open and receptive of ideas and to be supportive of those who present their research . . . the intention was to look beyond and toward how the ideas and methods presented could be extended and/or strengthened in future research. To that end, Madeleine Leininger was charged to present the opening paper, *The Research Critique*. It was learned later . . . that several of those who would be presenting critiques later in the program disappeared to their rooms to rewrite portions of their critiques. We were on our way toward creating a climate that would lead to great things for nursing research in the West.

Five investigators, five critics, the planning committee and staff, and 44 participants attended that first conference in Salt Lake City. We all were novices in the research enterprise; only 20 of those at that conference had earned doctorates. Still, we felt an excitement about what we were accomplishing; we talked about the research we were doing, were starting, or would like to start. Little did we know that on that day 50 years ago the seeds that were being planted would grow into the Western Institute of Nursing conferences we now experience. But, as R. Maureen Maxwell said in her closing remarks at that first conference, "Research in nursing in the West will move on" (Maxwell, 1968a, p. 168). And it has done so.

Following the now-classic Keynote presentation, *The Research Critique: Nature, Function, and Art,* by Madeleine Leininger (see Leininger, 1968), the five presenters gave their presentations with professional critique. These are shown in Table 2-1 (adapted from Murphy, 1992, p. 40).

Table 2-1. Research Presentations – First Communicating Nursing Research Conference	
Marian Olson University of Hawaii (Olson, 1968) Dorothy E. Johnson, Critique University of California Los Angeles (Wayne, 2014)	Social Influences on Student Nurses in Their Choice of Ideal and Practiced Solutions to Nursing Problems
Jacqueline L. Holt [Vandemann] University of Washington (M. V. Batey & P. McNeil, personal communication, September 22, 2016) Helen H. Schuster, Critique Anthropology University of Wyoming (P. McNeil, personal communication, September 22, 2016)	Discussion of the Method and the Clinical Implications from the Study: Children's Recall of a Preschool Age Hospital Experience After an Interval of Five Years
L. Frances Pride Columbia Union College Takoma Park, MD (later changed to Washington Adventist University (P. McNeil, personal communication, September 22, 2016) Louise W. Mansfield, Critique University of Washington (P. McNeil, personal communication, September 22, 2016)	An Experimental Study of the Effect of an Interpersonal Nursing Approach on an Adrenal Stress Index in Hospitalized Medical Patients
Ada Sue Hinshaw University of California San Francisco (M. V. Batey, personal communication, October 30, 2016) Gladys Sorensen, Critique University of Arizona (Prabook, 2016)	Effects of Teacher and Situational Variables on Student Achievement: An Example of Action Research
Juanita F. Murphy Arizona State University (Jackson, 2016) Betty Mitsunaga, Critique University of Colorado University of Washington (WINb, 2015).	Psychiatric Nurses and Their Patients: A Study of Role Perceptions and Performance

Second and Third Conferences: Back to Utah
   1969: *Problem Identification and the Research Design* and
   1970: *Methodological Issues in Research*

From 1962 and 1964 through 1970, Utah was represented by at least one member of the WCHEN Executive Committee (Mildred Quinn as Chair, Genee Van Sant, and Verle Lesnan from the University of Utah; and Ruth Swenson from Weber State College), which might have offered one factor in the selection of the location of Salt Lake City for the first three conferences. Or, perhaps it might have been simply a geographically "central" location in the West (WIN, 2007).

The format of the second conference generally followed that of the first one, with the addition of formal responses to critique by the research presenters. The conference was opened by remarks by R. Maureen Maxwell and a keynote by Katherine Hoffman, followed by research presentations from Ellamae Branstetter, with critique by Madeleine Leininger; Marjorie Batey, with critique by Marlene Kramer; Mary Patterson, with critique by Janelle Krueger; Margaret Spaulding, with general discussion critique due to the illness of planned critique by Imogene Cahill; Lois Johns, with critique by Patricia Hummel, Margaret Berry, and Eugene Levine. The conference ended with responses and views of the future by Anne Davis and R. Maureen Maxwell.

Batey (1992, p. 55) shared some of the drama behind the scenes in producing the second conference and its proceedings: a reminder of the technical challenges of the early times:

> No, everything does not go as smoothly as the printed proceedings would suggest. The "incinerator project" (Volume 2, 1969) is a dramatic case in point. I had done my part of the work on Volume 1 while in Boulder as a member of the WCHEN staff. As I completed a paper, I walked it down the hall to Lee's [Lee Gladish, staff member responsible for all publications from WICHE (M. V. Batey, personal communication January 18, 2017)] office so he could move on his effort on the same paper. By the time of Volume 2 work, I was in Seattle. Technology was relatively limited: a long carriage typewriter, carbon paper and tape for ease of cut and paste were the readily available tools. Certainly, photocopy was available, but was costly and was not used extensively. As I completed work on the papers, I mailed the completed work to Lee. One day after all papers were completed, Lee called me. In his gentle voice, he asked if I had the copy of one of the papers. "No, Lee, I sent them all to you." He ignored my answer and asked about another paper, and then yet another. I was getting more irritable with each request and finally asked, "What did you do, lose them all?" Still in his quiet, gentle voice, he answered, "Yes." The previous evening he had completed putting everything in readiness for the printer [note that then a "printer" was a place of business with printing machines—not an extension of a computer], but the print shop was closed. He returned to his office the next morning to take the papers to the printer, and they were no place to be found. We never discovered what happened to the original papers! Each author was contacted for another copy of the presented paper. Some had retained true copies, some had only drafts . . . Yes, we did manage to reconstruct the proceedings, but it took more than a lost summer to do so.

The third conference in Salt Lake City brought a new WCHEN Executive Committee Chair, Kathryn Smith from the University of Colorado. New members, Marjorie Batey and Jeanne Quint (Benoliel) from the University of Washington, officially joined Kathryn Hoffman and R. Maureen Maxwell on the Conference Planning Committee (WIN, 1992, p. 394). Marjorie Batey gave the Keynote Address. The conference in 1970 marked the first research presentations by more than one author: "Change in Problem-solving Ability Among Nurses Receiving Mental Health Consultation: A Pilot Study" by Grace Wiest Deloughery, Betty Newman, and Kristine Gebbie; and "Effect of Postoperative Recovery Rate and Comfort of Four Approaches to Nursing Care of Dogs: A Pilot Study" by Betty Jo Hadley, Margaret Berry, and Margaret Kaufmann (see Batey, 1970). The tradition continued of a formal critique following each presentation.

Fourth and Fifth Conferences: On to Nevada
1971: *Is the Gap Being Bridged?* and
1972: *The Many Sources of Nursing Knowledge*
The next two conferences were held in the state of Nevada. The fourth conference, *Is the Gap Being Bridged?* was held in Las Vegas in 1971; and the fifth conference, *The Many Sources of Nursing Knowledge,* was in Reno in the next year. By the fourth conference, "Research Clinics" were added as consulting sessions, mock reviews, and/or discussion groups to help new investigators translate concepts to proposals, to exchange ideas to advance lines of inquiry, and to inform each other of research in progress (Batey, 1973a; Benoliel, 1973). Batey (1973b, p. 216 explained:

> The Clinic was conceived of as a group of scholars discussing a study under development for the purposes of 1) contributing through their collective insights to the sound development of a given study, and 2) highlighting issues in design which would bear also upon their present and future research.

These clinics were called "innovative" by federal officers. Doris Bloch, then Chief of the Research Grants Section of the Nursing Research Branch, Division of Nursing, Public Health Service, even attended a mock review at one of the clinics (Gortner, 1992, p. 64). Note that neither the National Center for Nursing Research, established in 1986, nor the National Institute of Nursing Research, which came in 1993 (NIH, 2016), were even a thought at the time.

In the Keynote Address, R. Maureen Maxwell reported that in the 1950s, there were only 20 nurses with doctorates in the West, by 1965 there were 50 nurses with doctorates, and by this year of 1972, there were approximately 75 nurses with doctorates in the West (Maxwell, 1972, p. 1). Another highlight of the conference in 1972 was the growing range of methods reported in nursing research, with one qualitative exemplar by Agnes Aamodt, "The Child View of Health and Healing," that featured analysis of children's drawings (see Aamodt, 1972).

Dorothy McLeod, one of the first two faculty members to establish the school of nursing at Arizona State University (ASU, 2016) replaced Katherine Hoffman on the Conference Planning Committee. Marjorie Batey, Jeanne Benoliel, and R. Maureen Maxwell continued on the committee through the fourth and fifth conferences. Gladys Sorensen was Chair of the WCHEN Executive Committee (WIN, 1992, p. 394).

Arizona in 1973: *Collaboration and Competition in Nursing Research*

The Conference Planning Committee for the sixth conference included Marjorie Batey, Jeanne Benoliel, R. Maureen Maxwell, Dorothy McLeod, and the addition of Dorothy Martin from Loma Linda University. Ellamae Branstetter, from Arizona State University, was Chair of the WCHEN Executive Committee (WIN, 1992, p. 395). At this conference, the "research brief" was added to highlight "studies relatively circumscribed in scope" but worthy of discussion to advance the science (Batey, 1973b, p. 216). Jeanne Benoliel (1973, p. 8) offered the Keynote message, confirming the need for exchange of ideas in a spirit of "competition and collaboration," underscoring the value of the annual conference, noting that "the spread of knowledge requires people who are willing to exchange their ideas and to barter in the marketplace of concepts and constructs and theories."

The format had expanded slightly to include more papers, without the formal critique presentation of each project. The nature of the research seemed to mature, shown by increased reference to conceptual frameworks and refined methods (see Batey, 1973a).

The conference in Phoenix was the last of the series of six to be funded by the Division of Nursing. There were clear indications that the series had been highly successful, with high interest from organization members. The quality of the research presentations continued to improve, "and the level of the discussion among the participants showed increased research sophistication but with an amiable respect for different modes of inquiry" (Gortner, 1992, p. 64). The conference had become a significant part of the mission and activities of WCHEN. But, funding from the federal Division of Nursing was no longer available. Federal politics had changed over the years of the administration of President Richard Nixon, and priorities among federal funding sources for nursing and/or research were not the same as they had been when the conference had been originally funded (see McAthie, 1992, p. 75). No solutions for support emerged during the conference.

The Western Society for Research in Nursing (WSRN)

By the next semi-annual meeting of the WCHEN Council in October, 1973, the continuation of the conference was the critical issue. According to the Chair of the Executive Committee, Ellamae Branstetter (1992; WIN, 2016c), Jo Eleanor Elliott suggested three funding options: (1) conduct smaller conferences throughout the region under an existing WCHEN funded project, (2) develop a self-supporting annual conference, or (3) attempt the submission of another proposal for federal funding (WCHEN, 1973). A special executive session met with representatives of the Division of Nursing on the evening before the General Business Meeting of the Council. Present at that meeting were Executive Committee members Branstetter, Sister Eleanor Francis, Elda Popiel, and Anna Shannon; Jo Eleanor Elliott and WCHEN staff; and federal representatives, Jessie Scott, Executive Director of the Division of Nursing and Assistant Surgeon General, U. S. Public Health Service and consultants, Mary Lou McAthie and Elinor Stanford. The federal representatives confirmed that continued funding was not an option. The entire group decided to take the risk to propose a plan for a self-supporting organization to continue the conference. Mary Lou McAthie suggested the name of "Western Society for Research in Nursing." The decision was presented to the WCHEN General Assembly for vote, which was overwhelming in support, and WSRN was born! (Branstetter, 1992).

The official proposal for the new organization outlined WSRN as a component of the existing WCHEN enterprise, annual individual membership, continuation of the annual *Communicating Nursing Research* conference with attendance registration fees (funding to participants had been provided in the past), formation of an official Conference Planning Committee, and provision of staff support by WCHEN. Funding support was begun immediately by the offer of founding memberships at $25 (Approximate value of $179 in 2016 [see *Dollar Times,* 2016; *Saving.Org*, 2016]). Participants who came forth with the dues were given an official numbered certificate noting their founding membership (McAthie, 1992). Members scrambled for the lowest number to be founding member number one, or two, or three, etc. Branstetter (1992, p. 70) noted, "There was a great clamor among the group, as each tried to produce the first check in order to be Founding Member *number one*" (Branstetter, 1992, p. 70). McAthie (1992, p. 76) confirmed, ". . . the conference attendees became unruly immediately after the vote was taken . . . there was a great, confusing scramble to be first to pay the twenty-five dollar dues. Everyone wanted to be first."

Though the representatives from the federal Division of Nursing may not have been able to offer funding, they were certainly personally engaged in the plan. Indeed, the scuffle over who could be the first founding member of WSRN was between them: Marylou McAthie, who is credited with originating the name for the organization, and Elinor Stanford, who eventually claimed the title of "Founder Number One." Eventually, it was resolved with McAthie honored as "Founder Number Zero" (Branstetter, 1992; McAthie, 1992).

And so, again, a small group of courageous pioneers advanced the cause for nursing research in the West. Who were these people? Ellamae Branstetter was the youngest of a family of eight, born in Miami, Oklahoma, and raised in the Midwest. She graduated from nursing school at Jewish Hospital in St. Louis in 1944 and earned the B.S. from St. Louis University, M.P.H. from the University of Minnesota, and the Ph.D. from the University of Chicago in 1969. In 1958, she was recruited to the Visiting Nursing Service in Phoenix, and helped to begin the nursing program at Arizona State University (ASU) as one of its three first faculty members. Following a brief absence from ASU, she returned to establish its first graduate program in nursing. She was a pioneer proponent of nurse practitioner practice and nurse-managed clinics. She died at the age of 90 in 2013 after a lifetime of service to nursing in the West and garnering many awards in teaching and research (*Arizona Republic*, 2013; Stevenson, 2007).

Also born and educated in the Midwest, Sister Eleanor Francis served as a psychiatric nurse, nurse educator, and hospital chaplain. She worked in several hospitals and schools of nursing in Nebraska, at the University of New Mexico, and eventually as a hospital chaplain at St. Francis Hospital in Colorado Springs, where she died at the age of 94 in 2014 (*The Gazette*, 2014).

Elda S. Popiel came from Kansas to the University of Colorado to earn a doctoral degree. She became involved in continuing education, and stayed in the West. She was among the original members of the Continuing Education Seminar of WCHEN, and responsible for several leadership courses funded by the Kellogg Foundation through WCHEN. She proclaimed that WCHEN was "the biggest influence" on continuing education in nursing in the state of Colorado, and eventually became known herself as a "mother of continuing education" (Yoder-Wise, 1983; 1994). She served as Assistant

Dean for Continuing Education in Nursing at the University of Colorado for 18 years. She was also among the pioneers who established the Council on Continuing Education and Staff Development of the American Nurses Association, was the associate editor of the *Journal of Continuing Education in Nursing* (Yoder-Wise, 1994), and is listed among the WIN Emeriti (WIN, 2015b).

Anna M. Shannon is well-known as an institution within the WCHEN/WIN community in the West. She was a strong proponent of the success of the structure and resources of the organization (see Shannon, 1992). She was the first recipient of the WIN Jo Eleanor Elliott Leadership Award (WIN, 2007, p. 56) and in the first group to be inducted into the Western Academy of Nurses (see Appendix E). She served as elected Chair of WCHEN in 1984 (2016c). Among the most impressive descriptions of her influence comes from her niece, Sarah Shannon, who is currently the Senior Associate Dean for Academic Affairs at Oregon Health and Science University (OHSU, 2016) (see Note 2-A):

> The first [person of inspiration] is my aunt, Dr. Anna M. Shannon. Anna is a nationally-known leader in nursing education, a beloved former Dean of Montana State University, and a respected pioneer in nursing leadership. The mentorship award, which is given annually at the Western Institute of Nursing spring meeting is named in her honor . . . She invested her energy and attention in each of us by guiding us to think about who we were and who we wanted to become. [She] continues to live in Bozeman, Montana and I visit her as often as possible to soak up her wisdom and share our mutual love of the Big Sky State.

The WIN *Anna M. Shannon Mentorship Award* was created in her honor by Kathleen Long and Jeanne Kearns "for her unselfish efforts to support and promote the professional growth of other nurses in the West" (WIN, 2016b). To date, 26 outstanding mentors from nine states have received the award.

The federal Division of Nursing was represented by three pioneers, who, though they could not assure funding, were supportive of the vision and work of WSRN. Jessie Scott graduated from Wilkes-Barre General Hospital School of Nursing in Pennsylvania, earned the bachelor's degree in nursing from the University of Pennsylvania, master's degree in personnel administration from Columbia University, and then served as assistant executive secretary of the Pennsylvania Nurses Association until she entered the United States Public Health Service in 1955, eventually promoted to Rear Admiral. In 1957, she was appointed deputy chief of the service, and in 1964 was appointed second director of nursing under the Surgeon General. She was also President of the Commission on Graduates of Foreign Nursing Schools. She was later awarded the Distinguished Service Medal by the Department of Health, Education, and Welfare, was named a "living legend" by the American Academy of Nursing (ANA, 2014; Sullivan, 2009), and honored with an award by the American Nurses Association in her name (ANA, 2016).

Marylou McAthie began her career at the Presbyterian School of Nursing in Chicago. She held nursing positions at Oak Park Hospital in Illinois, Sacramento State University, and San Joaquin General Hospital before joining the United States Public Health Service. She consulted to American Samoa, Guam, Palau, Micronesia, and the

Marshall Islands, and helped to establish the American Pacific Nursing Leadership Council. Following her federal service, she joined the faculty at Sonoma State University in Rohnert Park, California; and continued as a local and national leader and supporter of WIN and WSRN (*Press Democrat*, 2013; SSU, 2016). Sonoma State University continues to honor her with emerita status (SSU, 2014; SSU, 2016, p. 59).

Elinor Stanford was born in Springfield, Massachusetts and graduated from Springfield Hospital School of Nursing. She earned a bachelor's degree in nursing from Boston University, a master's from Catholic University of America, and completed doctoral courses in education at Boston University. Before joining the United States Public Health Service, she served as a Nurse Consultant for the Agency for International Development in the Philippines and for several hospitals and schools of nursing in Massachusetts. She was Acting Director of the Division of Nursing from 1979 to 1980 and Deputy Director from 1975 to 1982. She retired at the rank of Captain after more than 30 years of federal service (*Washington Post*, 2011).

Following the formality of approval of the Western Society for Research in Nursing by WICHE early in 1974, WSRN was officially established. The *Communicating Nursing Research* conference continued without interruption from its first vision, now ostensibly self-supported by memberships and registration fees, and an integral part of WCHEN. By the time of its official recognition, 147 founding members went on record to extend its vision (Branstetter, 1992).

Marjorie Batey (1975, p. iii) reflected the general sentiment of pioneer nurses in the West:

When the series was launched in 1968, it seemed a Utopian dream that such a commitment to provide a continuing forum for nursing research should be realized in such a relatively short time.

WSRN provided a structure within WIN to focus on the development and dissemination of research and promotion of the continuing unique professional collegiality among nurses in the West. It represented growth and a new foundation to advance the improvement of health care as the mission of the discipline.

References

Aamodt, A. (1972). The child view of health and healing. In M. V. Batey (Ed.), *Communicating Nursing Research, 5* (pp. 38-54). Boulder, CO: WCHEN.

American Nurses Association (ANA). (2014). RADM Jessie M. Scott, DSc, RN, FAAN (1915-2009) (2014 inductee). *Hall of fame.* Retrieved September 21, 2016 from http://www.nursingworld.org/FunctionalMenuCategories/AboutANA/Honoring-Nurses/NationalAwardsProgram/HallofFame/2014-HOF-Inductees/Jessie-M-Scott-2014.html.

American Nurses Association (ANA). (2016). Jessie M. Scott award. Retrieved September 21, 2016 from http://www.nursingworld.org/DocumentVault/Awards/Jessie-M-Scott-.pdf.

Arizona Republic. (2013, May 9). Obituary: Ellamae Branstetter. Retrieved September 17, 2016 from http://www.legacy.com/obituaries/azcentral/obituary.aspx?pid=164699211.

Arizona State University College of Nursing (ASU). (2016). College timeline. Retrieved September 15, 2016 from https://nursingandhealth.asu.edu/about/college-timeline.

Batey, M. V. (Ed.) (1968). *Communicating Nursing Research, 1.* Boulder, CO: WCHEN.

Batey, M. V. (1968) Preface. In M. V. Batey (Ed.), *Communicating Nursing Research, 1* (pp. v-vi). Boulder, CO: WCHEN.

Batey, M. V. (Ed.) (1970). *Communicating Nursing Research, 3.* Boulder, CO: WCHEN.

Batey, M. V. (Ed.). (1973a). *Communicating Nursing Research, 6.* Boulder, CO: WCHEN.

Batey, M. V. (1973b). Reflections – and the way ahead. In M. V. Batey (Ed.), *Communicating Nursing Research, 6* (pp. 215-221). Boulder, CO: WCHEN.

Batey, M. V. (1975). Foreword. In M. V. Batey (Ed.), *Communicating Nursing Research, 7* (p. iii). Boulder, CO: WCHEN.

Batey, M. V. (1992). Communicating nursing research: The conference proceedings—early years (AKA: My ten lost summers). In *The anniversary book: A history of nursing in the west 1956-1992* (pp. 51-56). Boulder, CO: WIN.

Benoliel, J. Q. (1973). Collaboration and competition in nursing research. In M. V. Batey (Ed.), *Communicating Nursing Research, 6* (pp. 1-11). Boulder, CO: WCHEN.

Benoliel, J. Q. (1992). The changing climate of WSRN conferences. In *The anniversary book: A history of nursing in the West 1956-1992* (pp. 125-129). Boulder, CO: WIN.

Branstetter, E. (1992). The Western Society for Nursing Research begins. In *The anniversary book: A history of nursing in the West 1956-1992* (pp. 69-73). Boulder, CO: WIN.

Brink, P. J. (1992). The *Western Journal of Nursing Research.* In *The anniversary book: A history of nursing in the West 1956-1992* (pp. 57-61). Boulder, CO: WIN.

Clayton, B. (2000). Mildred Dericott [sic] Rordame Quinn: 1908-1989. In V. L. Bullough & L. Sents, L., Eds., *American nursing: A biographical dictionary* (pp. 237-240). New York City, NY: Springer.

Deseret News (2000, January 12). Obituary: Mildred Derricott Rordame Quinn. Retrieved January 16, 2017 from http://www.deseretnews.com/article/738017/Obituary-Mildred-Derricott-Rordame-Quinn.html?pg=all.

Dollar Times (2016). Inflation calculator. Retrieved September 19, 2016 from http://www.dollartimes.com/inflation/inflation.php?amount=25&year=1973.

Editorial (1965). The first American Nurses Association nursing research conference. *Nursing Research, 14(2),* 99.

Elliott, J. E. (1968). Developmental background of the project. In M. Batey, Ed., *Communicating Nursing Research, 1* (pp. 9-12). Boulder, CO: WCHEN.

Elliott, J. E. (1990). Nursing research: Transcending the 20th century. In *Communicating Nursing Research, 23* (pp. 3-7). Boulder, CO: WIN.

Elliott, J. E. (1992). The West's regional efforts in nursing research. In *The anniversary book: A history of nursing in the West 1956-1992* (pp. 25-30). Boulder, CO: WIN.

Gortner, S. (1992). The Federal role. In *The anniversary book: A history of nursing in the West 1956-1992* (pp. 63-67). Boulder, CO: WIN.

Jackson, J. (2016, May 17). New book tackles lives of caregivers. *The Daily Courier.* Retrieved September 14, 2016 from http://www.dcourier.com/news/2016/may/17/column-new-book-tackles-lives-caregivers/.

Johnson, J. (2012, December 30). Madeleine Leininger: A great woman with a great story. *Sutton Nebraska Museum.* Sutton, NE: Sutton Historical Society. Retrieved September 10, 2016 from http://wuttonhistoricalsociety.blogspot.com/2012/12/madeleine-leininger-great-woman-with.htm.

King, I. (1968). Toward the future in nursing research. In M. V. Batey (Ed), *Communicating Nursing Research, 1* (pp. 158-166). Boulder, CO: WCHEN.

King, I. M. (1971). *Toward a theory for nursing.* Hoboken, NJ: John Wiley & Sons.

Leininger, M. M. (1968). The research critique: Nature, function, and art. In M. V. Batey (Ed.), *Communicating Nursing Research, 1* (pp. 20-32). Boulder, CO: WCHEN.

Maxwell, R. M. (1968a). Concluding comments. In M. V. Batey (Ed.), *Communicating Nursing Research, 1* (pp. 167-168). Boulder, CO: WCHEN.

Maxwell, R. M. (1968b). The preparation of teachers of nursing. *Nursing Forum, 7(4),* 365-374.

Maxwell, R. M. (1972). The many sources of nursing knowledge. In M. V. Batey (Ed.), *Communicating Nursing Research, 5* (pp. 1-8). Boulder, CO: WCHEN.

McAthie, M. (1992). The Western Society for Research in Nursing: How it started. In *The anniversary book: A history of nursing in the West 1956-1992* (pp. 75-78). Boulder, CO: WIN.

Murphy, J. F. (1992). The first nursing research conference in the West. In *The anniversary book: A history of nursing in the West 1956-1992* (pp. 37-42). Boulder, CO: WIN.

National Institutes of Health (NIH). (2016). Important events in the National Institute of Nursing Research history. Retrieved September 17, 2016 from https://www.ninr.nih.gov/aboutninr/history#.V93Dy63RvuY.

Nurse.com. (2012, August). *Nursing visionary Madeleine Leininger dies at 87.* Retrieved January 16, 2017 from https://www.nurse.com/blog/2012/08/17/nursing-visionary-madeleine-leininger-dies-at-87/.

Olson, M. E. (1968). Comparison of head nurse and staff nurse attitudes toward various aspects of nursing care. *Nursing Research, 17(4),* 349-352.

Oregon Health and Science University (OHSU). (2016, September 7). Q and A with Dr. Shannon, senior associate dean for academic affairs. Retrieved September 17, 2016 from http://www.ohsu.edu/xd/education/schools/school-of-nursing/about/news-events/q-a-shannon.cfm.

Prabook. (2016). Gladys Elaine Sorensen. Retrieved September 14, 2016 from http://prabook.com/web/person-view.html?profileId=87399.

Press Democrat. (2013, January 31 to February 1). Obituary: Marylou McAthie. Retrieved September 21, 2016 from http://www.legacy.com/obituaries/ pressdemocrat/obituary-print.asp...

Saving.Org (2016). Value of $25 in 1973. Retrieved September 19, 2016 from http:// www.saving.org/inflation/inflation.php?amount=25&year=1973.

Shannon, A. M. (1992). WSRN as a society within WIN or WSRN within WCHEN. WIN: A nested, repeated measures design. In *The anniversary book: A history of nursing in the West 1956-1992* (pp. 133-134). Boulder, CO: WIN.

Sonoma State University (SSU). (2014, May 10). Commencement. Rohnert Park, CA: SSU. Retrieved September 21, 2016 from http://www.sonoma.edu/uaffairs/ commencement/images/2014-SSU-commencement-program.

Sonoma State University (SSU). (2016, January 4). In Memoria: SSU Emeritus and Retired Faculty and Staff Association. Retrieved September 21, 2016 from http://www.sonoma.edu/erfa/memoriam.html.

Stevenson, P. (2007, January 29). Ellamae Branstetter recalls starting the nurse practitioner program and the first nursing clinic for ASU. ASU Retirees Association, Arizona State University. Retrieved September 17, 2016 from https://asura.asu.edu/BranstetterVideoClip.

Sullivan, P. (2009, October 30). Public health official promoted nurse training. *Washington Post.* Retrieved September 21, 2016 from http://www.washingtonpost. com/wp-dyn/content/article/2009/10/29/AR2009102904545_pf.html.

Tampa Bay Times. (2007, December 28). Obituary: Imogene M. King. Retrieved January 16, 2017 from http://www.legacy.com/obituaries/sptimes/obituary. aspx?pid=100288228.

The Gazette. (2014, December 3). Obituary: Eleanor Hemmer OSF. Retrieved September 17, 2016 from http://www.legacy.com/obituaries/gazette/obituary. aspx?n=eleanor-hemmer&pid=173352948&.

University of Nebraska Medical Center (UNMC). (2012, August 14). Legendary nurse, Madeleine Leininger, PhD., dies at 87. *Breakthroughs for life.* Omaha, NE: UNMC. Retrieved September 10, 2016 from http://app1.unmc.edu/PublicAffairs/ TodaySite/sitefiles/today_full_pr...

Visionary Madeleine Leininger dies at 87. (2012, August 17). Retrieved September 10, 2016 from https://www.nurse.com/blog/2012/08/17/nursing-visionary- nadeleine-leininger-dies-at-87/.

Washington Post. (2011, August 26 - August 28). Death notice: Elinor D. Stanford. Retrieved September 21, 2016 from http://www.legacy.com/obituaries/ washingtonpost/obituary-print.asp...

Washington State Nurses Association (WSNA). (2004). Marjorie Batey. *WSNA hall of fame.* Retrieved September 10, 2016 from https://www.wsna.org/hall0of- fame/2004/marjorie-batey.

Wayne, G. (2014). Dorothy E. Johnson: Pioneer of behavioral system model. *Nurselabs.* Retrieved September 14, 2016 from http://nurseslabs.com/dorothy-e-johnson/.

Western Council on Higher Education for Nursing (WCHEN). (1973, June 27-28). *Minutes, executive committee.* Boulder, CO: WCHEN.

Western Institute of Nursing (WIN). (2007). *The anniversary book: 50 years of advancing nursing in the West.* Portland, OR: WIN.

Western Institute of Nursing (WIN). (2015b). WIN Emeriti. Retrieved September 14, 2016 from http://winursing.org/?query=WIN+Emeriti.

Western Institute of Nursing (WIN). (2016a). About WIN. Retrieved January 16, 2017 from https://www.winursing.org/about-win/.

Western Institute of Nursing (WIN). (2016b). Anna M. Shannon mentorship award. Retrieved January 21, 2017 from https://www.winursing.org/anna-m-shannon-mentorship-award/.

Western Institute of Nursing (WIN). (2016c, January 11, 2016). History subcommittee: Potential interviewees for the 50th anniversary project. WIN Archives, Portland, OR.

Yoder-Wise, P. S. (1983). Living history series: Elda S. Popiel. *The Journal of Continuing Education in Nursing, 14(6),* 27-30. Retrieved September 17, 2016 from http://www.healio.com/nursing/journals/jcen/1983-11-14-6/%7Ba5dfcd13-f47d-483f-8c06-bc87a64b8ed9%7D/living-history-series-elda-s-popiel.

Yoder-Wise, P. S. (1994). A tribute to Elda S. Popiel (1912-1994). *The Journal of Continuing Education in Nursing, 25(6),* 245. Retrieved September 17, 2016 from http://www.healio.com/nursing/journals/jcen/1994-11-25-6/%7B2fd69f33-738a-4f2b-b391-9fbfb83102af%7D/a-tribute-to-elda-popiel-rn-msn-1912-1994.

Notes

2-A. Unless there is a compelling reason in an archival or published source, in this document OHSU will be called by its current title, Oregon Health and Science University.

Chapter Three

Communicating Nursing Research, 1974-1985:
"EXPERIMENTATION AND CHANGE" AND "CHANGING OF THE GUARD"

Chapter Three
Communicating Nursing Research, 1974-1985: "EXPERIMENTATION AND CHANGE" AND "CHANGING OF THE GUARD"

Benoliel (1992) referred to the first five years of the Western Society for Research in Nursing (WSRN) of the Western Council on Higher Education for Nursing (WCHEN) as a time of "Experimentation and Change," reflecting the transition and early development of the organization and the conference. The end of federal funding, which had allowed for financially hosting invited participants (Benoliel, 1992; Mitsunaga, 1992), marked a new era that required mechanisms for support and new structures for the conference. The "grand experiment" of a self-supporting conference "became the model for other research conferences in the country" (Shannon, 1992, p. 133). Shannon noted that "WCHEN created WSRN," and that "the support given WSRN by [WCHEN]/ WIN is so obvious as to be invisible" (Shannon, 1992, pp. 133-134). She warned that the *Communicating Nursing Research* conference was not totally financially self-sufficient or totally independent of the greater organization of WCHEN. She was a continuing advocate for support by members of WCHEN/WIN for the benefit of the research conference.

With the advent of WSRN, the structure of WCHEN was changed to create a different composition of the Executive Board and the addition of steering committees over specific nursing issues. Marjorie Dunlap, from the University of California San Francisco, was elected Chair of the Executive Board (WIN, 1992, p. 395). The Board outlined a five-year plan with twenty goals, many of which addressed needs for increased research, especially related to clinical applications, as well as research dissemination under WSRN and the *Communicating Nursing Research* conference (WIN, 1992, p. 12).

A Foundation for Continuing Development of Researchers in the West
Concurrent with the beginnings of the conference was the wise attention to continuing development of nurse researchers, regional research teams, and promoting the growth of promising research projects. One example was the project by Janelle Krueger and Allen Nelson to survey regional needs for research support and doctoral prepared faculty (see Krueger & Nelson, 1977).

Carol Lindeman also advised, guided, and led several important initiatives at WCHEN. One significant example is the WICHE Regional Program for Nursing Research Development, funded by the Division of Nursing from 1971 to 1978. Principal Investigators included Jean Berthold (1971-1973), Carol Lindeman (1973-1976), and Janelle Krueger (1976-1978) (Krueger, 1992). Others who made significant contributions were Jo Eleanor Elliott, Mary Opal Wolanin, Allen Nelson, Vi Nielsen, Edith Modafferi, Marylou MacAthie, Hazel Chiffer, Bernice Szukalla, and Juanita Tate (Krueger, 1992). The project offered workshops for promising researchers who were convened in workgroups for specific consultation. Lindeman (1992, p. 90) described the project:

> The first workshop of promising nurses with promising research ideas included 16 nurses from clinical settings and 11 nurses from academic settings. Five states were represented. Throughout the six years of the grant, 289 nurses participated in these research workgroups . . . These

nurses came from 185 agencies, from all 13 Western states. More than 50% of the groups finished their work by the end of the grant . . . Twenty-six research proposals were submitted, ten were funded. Numerous publications were generated from the research. The impact of the program on individuals, patient care, and agencies was considerable.

In the continuation phases of the project, from 1974 to 1977, a more targeted approach produced 14 workgroups that focused on research development on topics related to quality of patient care. Success in funding and completed projects was impressive (Lindeman, 1992). Anna Shannon noted the success of this ambitious program enabled "hundreds of nurses" "to make contributions to research and see their contributions as valued and valuable. This effort produced both research conference presenters for the fledgling research conferences and an audience for these presentations" (Shannon, 1992, p. 133). This work also underscored focus and priority on quality of the *Communicating Nursing Research* conference from the beginning.

Also, in 1974, Carol Lindeman reported on a national Delphi survey of clinical nursing research priorities (see Lindeman, 1974). This confirmed an interest and perceived need for nursing to take leadership in research related to "professional relevance" and "social or patient welfare relevance," with priorities in areas of patient care, such as "nursing interventions related to stress, care of the aged, pain, and patient education" (Lindeman, 1974, p. 61).

Carol Ann Lehmann Lindeman grew up in the Midwest attending school in Racine, Wisconsin. She graduated from Deaconess Hospital School of Nursing in Milwaukee in 1955, chosen specifically because she "wanted to study where there were sick people." She earned B.S. and M.Ed. degrees from the University of Minnesota and the Ph.D. in educational psychology from the University of Wisconsin, Madison, following the assurance from the faculty that "they would not hold her nursing background against her." She taught nursing at St. Catherine's College in St. Paul, Minnesota and at the University of Wisconsin, Eau Claire. Lindeman served as Director of Nursing Research at Luther Hospital in Eau Claire. There, she developed an enduring philosophy that the best research is done when clinicians and academicians collaborate. Her work focused on nursing interventions and patient outcomes. She brought that experience to her successful work in Research Development at WCHEN (C. A. Lindeman, personal communication, January 11, 2017).

Lindeman served as Dean of the School of Nursing at Oregon Health and Science University from 1976 to 1995. She increased the number of advance practice nurses in the state and began the Ph.D. program in 1985. Her commitment to research as a key to excellence in education and practice was a hallmark of her tenure.

Throughout her administrative service, she continued her commitment to WCHEN/WIN. She was the last Chair of WCHEN and the first Chair of WIN. She keynoted the conference a record three times. The annual award to a New Researcher is named for her contributions. When the WIN headquarters moved from Colorado to Oregon, it was Dean Lindeman who offered space and support at no cost. Her influence in the discipline extends far beyond the West. Always with a focus on improvement of clinical practice (King & Lindeman, 1995), she has presented and consulted across the United States and Canada. She holds seven honorary degrees, and has served as President of Sigma Theta Tau International and President of the National League for Nursing (Ash & Weimer, 1998; Gaines, 2000; C. A. Lindeman, personal communication, January 11, 2017).

Evolving Format for the Conference

Under the leadership of Betty Mitsunaga, as the Chair of the Research Steering Committee within the new organizational structure, the format of the *Communicating Nursing Research* conference was changed, eliminating the formal critique of each presentation. The value of constructive critique was recognized, but some critiques had degenerated to become unfortunately "harsh and intimidating, rather than supportive and developmental" (Martin, 1992, p. 117) or even "mean spirited" (Shannon, 1992, p. 134). Further, it became more important to encourage higher participant attendance and a larger number of presentations to accommodate growing research in the region as well as to enhance financial stability of the conference. A new format was needed.

To San Francisco in 1974: *Critical Issues in Access to Data*

The Conference Planning Committee for the 1974 conference included Marjorie Batey and Jeanne Benoliel from the University of Washington, Dorothy McLeod from Arizona State University, and Dorothy Martin from Loma Linda University (WIN, 1992). Patricia MacElveen, from the University of Washington, delivered the Keynote Address. Eleven papers were presented to 99 participants in the new format that included groupings of papers into a symposium-like format with discussants replacing critiquers (Mitsunaga, 1992; Rawlinson, 1992). The new format was well received, and the conference seemed to be on its way toward a successful transition.

Directory of Research Instruments

Also begun in 1974 was the "ambitious project" to "compile a directory of instruments for nursing practice research." Carol Lindeman was the proposal writer and project director. Also involved were Mary Jane Ward and Doris Bloch as the federal contract officer (C. A. Lindeman, personal communication, October 24, 2016; see Ward, 1992), and Mark Fetler. The project included official advisory committees convening some of the finest researchers in the country: Marjorie Batey, University of Washington; Desmond Cartwright, University of Colorado College of Arts and Sciences; Gladys Courtney, University of Illinois; Rosemary Ellis, Case Western University; Elizabeth Hagen, Columbia University; Dorothy McLeod, Arizona State University; Claire Parsons, University of Virginia; Marjorie Dunlap, University of California; Kenneth Hopkins, University of Colorado School of Education; Alice Kuromoto, University of Washington; Barbara Mauger, Southern Regional Board of Education Department of Nursing Education; Barbara Stevens, Columbia University; Barbara Tate, University of Rhode Island; and Holly Wilson, University of California. They developed the famous two-volume *Blue Book*, that Susan Gortner called a "first generation publication in nursing research instrumentation" (Gortner, 1992, p. 65). The *Blue Book* was a landmark document and a significant resource to advance nursing research for many years.

1975: *Nursing Research Priorities: Choice or Chance* - Phoenix, Arizona and 1976: *Nursing Research in the Bicentennial Year* - Seattle, Washington

Personal tragedy marked the eighth conference with the loss of planning committee member, Dorothy Martin. She was killed in mid-air collision of her commuter plane to the Los Angeles airport as she was on her way to the planning meeting in Denver (Benoliel, 1992; Mitsunaga, 1992). The remaining bereaved planning committee members, Betty Mitsunaga, Janelle Kruger, and Gwen Stephens posed the conference title in honor of her memory (WIN, 1992, p. 396). Later, her message, "Variety of Sources of Nursing Research Data," was published posthumously.

Twenty-five studies were presented. Participants were more diverse, including "students, clinicians, and administrators" and an impressive number from outside the WCHEN region (Mitsunaga, 1992, p. 84). Dorothy McLeod, from Arizona State University, gave the Keynote message. The conference was financially solvent and the vision continued.

The ninth conference was planned by Chair Betty Mitsunaga, University of Washington; Susan Bradshaw, Los Angeles Southwest College; Pamela Brink, University of California Los Angeles; Dorothy Bloch, University of Colorado; Helen Bush, Arizona State University; and Ann Voda, University of Arizona (WIN, 1992, p. 396). Rheba de Tornyay, of the University of Washington and who advanced to national stature as an expert on nursing education, began the conference with the Keynote Address.

Third Executive Director of WICHE: Phillip Sirotkin
In 1976, Phillip Sirotkin became the Executive Director of WICHE. He came from the position of Executive Vice President at the State University of New York at Albany, though he had worked briefly with WICHE to organize the Mental Health program. Sirotkin was born in Moline, Illinois. He held degrees in political science from Wayne State University in Michigan and the University of Chicago. He had been a faculty member at Wellesley College, served in Army Intelligence in World War II, and worked as Executive Assistant to the Director of the California Department of Mental Hygiene and as Associate Director at the National Institute of Mental Health (MHEC, 2016).

Upon his arrival to WICHE, Sirotkin faced a variety of challenges, including serious budget shortfalls and threats of withdrawal from several states such as California, Wyoming, and Utah. Even as states found their own budget issues, Sirotkin significantly increased state membership fees (Abbott, 2004). He faced pressure from regional governors to "aggressively examine the WICHE mission and its related programs, projects, activities, and to take appropriate steps to strengthen WICHE management and WICHE's value to the states" (Abbott, 2004, p. 174). He acted by reducing WICHE staff, tightening travel policies, attempting to regionalize resources and graduate programs, and focusing on student exchange programs in medicine, dentistry, and veterinary medicine (Abbott, 2004). He was known as an effective political strategist and lobbyist. His focus was on improving access to professional education, allowing mostly medical and dental students who did not have programs in their home state to attend schools in other states in the region. He also instituted exchange programs for undergraduate students in the sciences (Culver, 2007). Sirotkin resigned from WICHE in 1989, and went on to establish the Midwestern Higher Education Compact, whose highest award still bears his name. At his retirement, he returned to Boulder, Colorado, his WICHE home. He died in 2007 (Culver, 2007; MHEC, 2016).

1977: *Optimizing Environments for Health: Nursing's Unique Perspective* - Denver, Colorado
The tenth anniversary of the *Communicating Nursing Research* conference was also the celebration of the 20th anniversary of WCHEN. The end of the first decade marked a significant step not only in the maturing of the conference, but in its

contribution to the discipline. Anyone who has ever served on the conference planning committee can witness that the planning discussions are among the most thoughtful, stimulating, and important professional conversations. It is where great minds of the discipline come together in an informal setting to consider the state of the science, dream, and plan a conference to advance that science. For example, Jean Lum (1992, p. 123) noted that the committees "continually explored new format[s]," such as inclusion of sessions with federal funding representatives, journal representatives, and published authors. She described the planning meetings as "stimulating, challenging, and sometimes agonizing debates over the selection of conference papers."

Occasionally, the fruits of these discussions truly advance the discipline to a better, higher level. This was especially true among the tenth group. The Research Steering Committee included Chair May Rawlinson from The University of Oregon Health Sciences Center; Dorothy Bloch from the University of Colorado; Susan Bradshaw from Los Angeles Southwest College; Pamela Brink from the University of California Los Angeles; Holly Wilson from California State College, Sonoma; Betty Mitsunaga from the University of Washington; and Sue Donaldson from the University of Washington (WIN, 1992, p. 397).

It is regrettable that no transcript exists of their planning meetings, but from their deliberations grew the idea for Sue Donaldson and Dorothy Crowley to offer the Keynote presentation on a theme of the unique perspective and science of nursing, "Discipline of Nursing: Structure and Relationship to Practice." The result was a seminal publication that continues to be a significant reference on the unique nature, science, and practice of nursing (see Donaldson & Crowley, 1978). Batey (1977, p. vii) immediately recognized the work as introducing "a new challenge and a new point of departure." And Rawlinson (1992, p. 110) observed, "This new challenge served to catapult us into the second decade." This confirms Batey's earlier note:

> Indeed, the theme of the entire conference was "to improve nursing practice through research . . . No longer was attention addressed only to nursing education. The WCHEN research function was interpreted as sharing research conducted on nursing questions, as critical appraisal of that research according to canons for truth, and as a forum for interchange among nurse investigators in academic and clinical settings in the western region. While the conferences varied somewhat from year to year, the guiding theme remained constant through the first six years (Batey, 1977, p. v-vi).

1978: *New Approaches to Communicating Nursing Research* - **Portland, Oregon**
Marion Schrum was the new Chair of the WCHEN Executive Board and the same planning committee continued (WIN, 1992, p. 397). Marjorie Batey returned to deliver the Keynote: "Research Communication: Its Functions, Audience, and Media." The eleventh conference, in 1978, indeed offered "new approaches to Communicating Nursing Research" by the introduction of poster sessions and symposia.

The poster sessions were conceived as an extension of the concept of the research clinics begun in 1971 to communicate, improve, and advance ongoing research (Rawlinson, 1992). But posters were not common at research conferences at the time, and the perceived risk was a possible reduction in the quality of the research or the presentation. But the potential benefit was to increase opportunities for participants to share their work, increase the number of participants, and thus increase conference revenue. The poster sessions allowed communication of research at different stages of the research and of the career of the researcher, provided a "training ground" for new researchers, encouraged professional socialization, and invited ongoing informal peer review at all stages of research (Rawlinson, 1992). Participation in poster sessions has continued to grow throughout the history of the conference. In 1978, 29 posters were exhibited, and by 2016, over 465 posters were presented, now with added judging and awards for outstanding research presentations in poster format (see WIN, 2016a).

The introduction of symposia was a step toward collaboration, communication among researchers with common research interests, a subtle step toward encouragement of a research program rather than individual studies, and toward building the science. In 1978, seven symposia were presented. That number has continued to grow, with as high as 24 symposia in 2013 and 2014 (WIN, 2013; 2014).

The first decade of the *Communicating Nursing Research* conference was a success that might have even exceeded expectations of the first visionary founders. The number of presentations had increased from five studies in 1968 to 17 podium, 7 symposia, and 29 poster in 1978.

The year 1978 also marked the establishment of the WCHEN New Researcher Award by Carol Lindeman to support nurse researchers early in their work. In 1987, its name was changed to recognize Lindeman as its founder (WIN, 1992, p. 13). As of 2017, 40 novice researchers from eight states have received the honor, and their addresses are published in each volume of *Communicating Nursing Research*. Evidence that the new researchers continue their commitment to research and to WIN is in their return to present at the conference. All but four have returned to present an average of four times (See Appendix C).

A Nursing Research Journal from the West
Pamela Brink (1992) has told the story of the beginning of a professional academic journal for nursing research. In 1978, a publisher editor contacted her with idea to develop a nursing journal, and sought her interest in becoming its editor. They were wide open on the type of nursing journal. She immediately proposed a research journal, pointing out that only one journal [*Nursing Research*] was devoted solely to research existed at the time. She shared the offer and her ideas with her colleagues at the next steering committee meeting of the Western Society for Research in Nursing (WSRN) (Brink, 1992, p. 57). It was at that fateful meeting that the title of the journal was born "in honor of a dream" of Katherine Hoffman: the *Western Journal of Nursing Research* (*WJNR*).

As she developed the format for the journal, Brink confirmed, "I wanted the major articles to be critiqued in print but also responded to by the author, just as in the early format in the *Communicating Nursing Research* issues" (Brink, 1992, p. 57). Confirming the value of the *people* in any story of pioneer events, she continued:

The idea was grand . . . I decided that since this was a "western" journal and since most of the ideas came from WCHEN, I would ask my colleagues to help me pull together and run the journal. So I looked for the people I respected and admired and who would have credibility in such an enterprise. I also wanted people who wanted to make a dream a reality (Brink, 1992, p. 58).

And so, the first masthead of the new journal featured an editorial board of pioneers from the West, shown in Table 3-1 (taken from Brink, 1992, p. 58).

Table 3-1 First Editorial Board of the *Western Journal of Nursing Research*

Editor: Pamela J. Brink (California)

Associate Editors

Jeanne Quint Benoliel (Washington)	Clinical Research
Rose McKay (Colorado)	Educational Research
Marilynn Wood (California)	General Research
Frank McLaughlin (California)	Information Exchange
Jeanne Kearns (WCHEN)	Regular Column
Mary Jane Amundson (Hawaii)	Regular Column

Department Editors

Marjorie Batey (Washington)	Technical Notes
Anne Davis (California)	Ethical Issues in Nursing Research
Ada Sue Hinshaw (Arizona)	Problems in Doing Nursing Research
Janelle Krueger (Arizona)	Using Research in Practice
Ruth Ludemann (Colorado)	Strategies for Teaching Nursing Research
Susan Gortner (California)	Researchmanship

Advisory Board (WSRN Steering Committee Members)

Ada Sue Hinshaw (Arizona)
Jean Lum (Hawaii)
Theresa Overfield (Utah)
May Rawlinson (Oregon)
Holly Wilson (California)

The *WJNR* began in 1979 with four issues a year as a collaborative project with WCHEN and KNI Publishing (S. T. Dearlove, personal communication, September 15, 2016). Through its early years of publication, the editorial board met at the annual *Communicating Nursing Research* conference, and for a time offered a 20 percent reduction in subscription rates to members of WSRN to "honor" its roots in WCHEN (Brink, 1992, p. 58). As the journal continued, distinguished researchers, mostly from the West, contributed as members of the editorial board, including Evelyn

Sobol, Nancy Fugate Woods, JoAnne Horsley, Toni Tripp-Reimer, Betty Chang, Olga Church, Marie Driever, Maryann Pranulis, and others. Also, over the years, the *Journal* published annual proceedings of WSRN, Keynote Addresses, New Researcher Award papers, and symposia (Brink, 1992). From 1981 to 1984, the journal published the total proceedings of the *Communicating Nursing Research* conference. By 1985, only the Keynote Addresses were regularly published (Kearns, 2003). In 1984, Sage Publishing acquired the *Journal.* By the year 2000, it had expanded to eight issues a year.

In 2003 the *Western Journal of Nursing Research* became the official journal of the Midwest Nursing Research Society, reflecting its importance to nursing research across the country. In 2007, Pamela Brink retired after 28 years of distinguished service, and Vicki Conn became the editor (S. T. Dearlove, personal communication, September 15, 2016). At that time, the tradition of critique of the published research reports was discontinued from the format of the journal (V. Conn, personal communication, September 29, 2016).

Brink (1992, p. 60, 61) noted:

Over the years I have been asked to consider a name change . . . that the title "Western" would "put off" readers and submitters but especially subscribers. In the beginning, I argued, "but the *New England Journal of Medicine* does not seem to have any difficulty with their regionalized name!" And I was told, "Yes, but they have been around a long time." My rejoinder has always been, "Well let's wait and see how long the *Western Journal of Nursing Research* will be around too. . . "

I still believe that the *WJNR* reflects a western spirit in that it has been pioneering in its approach to academic publishing. It developed a format copied by others; it has published materials others have emulated.

1979: *Credibility in Nursing Science* - Denver, Colorado
By 1979, WCHEN expanded its membership by inviting individuals and agencies in health care practice (WIN, 1992, p. 13). The first decade of success was noted by Keynote speaker, Susan Gortner (1979, p. 121), who referred to the conference format as "a model for the nation" and reported that the next American Nurses Association Council of Nursing Researchers would "emulate this model" (Rawlinson, 1992, p. 111). The new Research Steering Committee was chaired by Jean Lum, of the University of Hawaii, with members Ada Sue Hinshaw, University of Arizona; Theresa Overfield, Brigham Young University; May Rawlinson, University of Oregon Health Sciences Center; and Holly Wilson, who had moved to the University of California San Francisco (WIN, 1992, p. 398).

1980: *Directions for the 1980s* - Los Angeles, California and
1981: *Health Policy and Research* - Albuquerque, New Mexico
The new decade brought new opportunities for WCHEN's beloved leader, Jo Eleanor Elliott, as she became the Director of the Division of Nursing at the U.S. Department of Health and Human Services. Jeanne Kearns was immediately appointed Acting Director of the WICHE Nursing Program. Sally Ruybal then served a brief term as Director. Kearns then took the helm for the next 21 years (WIN, 1992, p. 14; WIN, 2007). Juanita Murphy, of Arizona State University, was Chair of the WCHEN

Executive Board, and Jean Lum continued to chair the WCHEN Research Steering Committee. Other committee members were Ada Sue Hinshaw and Theresa Overfield. New members were Clair Martin, University of Alaska; and Mary Quayhagen, University of Colorado (WIN, 1992, p. 398). In the 1980 Keynote, Carol Lindeman outlined the challenges for nursing research in the coming decade. In her Keynote in 1981, Betty Mitsunaga described the relationships among nursing knowledge, use of knowledge, and policy planning.

A New Executive Director for WCHEN: Jeanne Kearns

Jeanne Kearns grew up on Long Island, New York. She graduated from Lenox Hill Hospital School of Nursing in New York City. She earned the B.S. in nursing from Teachers College at Columbia University and the M.S. in nursing from Catholic University of America in Washington DC. Jeanne held faculty positions at the Lenox Hill School of Nursing and the College of Nursing at the Northeastern University in Boston. She then served as a Project Consultant at the Division of Nursing of the U. S. Public Health Service. Her work was to provide assistance to schools of nursing that were seeking funds under the federal Nurse Training Act of 1964. She later moved to Denver, Colorado to accept a faculty position at the University of Colorado. In 1975, Kearns joined the WICHE/WCHEN staff. That began what she calls "an exciting and meaningful professional life" (J. Kearns, personal communication, December 29, 2016). She was appointed Executive Director of WCHEN in 1982, where she served for 14 years. She secured funding for numerous projects and provided executive staff support for projects that continued to propel WCHEN as a significant force for the growth of professional nursing in the West. Perhaps her most significant contribution was her leadership in 1985-1986 in supporting the WCHEN Board of Governors, the second Committee of Seven, and the Expanded Committee of Seven through the difficult decision and implementation of the separation of WCHEN from WICHE to establish the autonomous and self-supporting organization of the Western Institute of Nursing (WIN). Her ability to work with diverse people in diverse circumstances was exactly what was needed in that transition. The executive headquarters of the new organization remained in the same WICHE building in Boulder, Colorado. In 1992, Kearns led the organization of WIN's 35th anniversary celebration (and the 25th anniversary of the *Communicating Nursing Research* conference), including the publication of *The Anniversary Book: A History of Nursing in the West 1956-1992* (WIN, 1992).

At the time of the retirement of Jeanne Kearns from WIN, the headquarters of the organization were moved from Colorado to the Oregon Health and Science University in Portland in 1996. In recognition for her service, Kearns was named to the Western Academy of Nurses and a WIN Emerita. She continues to contribute to WIN as needed, and openly expresses her fond memories and the impressive accomplishments of the organization (J. Kearns, personal communication, December 29, 2016). To this day, she continues to contribute to her community. For example, she was recently honored as an "Everyday Hero" by the local ABC television affiliate for her service as a volunteer for the last 20 years at the Denver Art Museum (Denver7, 2016).

"Changing of the Guard" and the Conference

Benoliel (1992, p. 127) referred to the early 1980s as the "Changing of the Guard." The themes and tone of the conference not only reflected the new leadership under Kearns, but "reflected the thinking of a new generation of investigator-scholars. The ideas showed a shift away from science as science and toward making nursing science visible to the public . . . research increased in sophistication of methods and sharpness of substantive focus. Isolated studies began to be replaced with presentations by research teams and multidisciplinary groups."

In 1980, Anna Shannon, from Montana State University, was the WCHEN Chair and Jean Lum, from the University of Hawaii, was Chair of the WCHEN Research Steering Committee. The Research Program Committee included Chair Clair Martin, University of Alaska; Betty Chang, University of California Los Angeles; Marjorie Crate Habeeb, University of San Francisco; Ann Muhlenkamp, Arizona State University; and Joan Shaver, University of Washington.

Carol Lindeman (1980) gave the Keynote Address in which she outlined five major challenges to advancing nursing research at the time:

1. Within the context of designing research, pursue the relationship between research problems and theory produced to increase the effectiveness of research efforts.
2. Systematize existing knowledge base in a science of nursing making the most effective use of our history.
3. Ensure that students are exposed to various theories and that they are challenged to critique and explore a variety of systematic formulations.
4. Facilitate career development of those who display creativity, a sense of inquiry, career commitment, scholarliness and respect for knowledge.
5. Create a reward system to enhance efforts to develop the science of nursing.

1982: *Nursing Science in Perspective* - Denver, Colorado
In 1982, reflecting recommendations of a task force, the original Charter of WCHEN was replaced by bylaws. Included in the new organizational documents was the Division of Affiliated Clinical Agencies to officially recognize membership and increase opportunities for nurses from clinical health care agencies that have worked with nursing education institutions (WIN, 1992, p. 13). Numbers of participants from clinical agencies have waxed and waned, with a continued general increase, across the years of the conference as indicated by participation in presentations and subsequent poster sessions. Those noteworthy agencies who have consistently participated in the conference are listed in Appendix F.

Kathryn Barnard, from the University of Washington, explored the cycle of research in nursing, practice in the profession, and maturing of the discipline. The mission to advance research to improve practice continued.

1983: *The Image of Nursing Research: Issues and Strategies* - Portland, Oregon
WCHEN Research Steering Committee again changed its name to the WCHEN Research Program Committee. Committee membership was Chair Clair Martin, University of Alaska; Betty Chang, University of California Los Angeles; Marjorie Habeeb, Hillhaven Convalescent Center, California; Ann Muhlenkamp, Arizona State University; Joan Shaver, University of Washington; and Anna Shannon, Montana State University (WIN, 1992, p. 399). Ada Sue Hinshaw opened the conference, focusing attention to the image of research in nursing.

Benoliel (1992, p. 127) reflected on a memorable example of the growing positive climate at the conference as they moved away from individual critique to group discussion and intellectual exchange, promoting "the usefulness of argument as a way of clarifying points of view yet respecting differences." It was a time in the general culture for advancing feminist theory, and the conference featured the symposium "Paradigm Change: New Perspectives for Nursing," at which a group from Utah made a case for the value of feminist inquiry, critical theory, and interpretive analysis for research in nursing." Benoliel remembered, "It was a provocative, informative, and highly crowded session."

RIFF-RAFF Breaks into 1983

In addition to conference presentations, symposia, and cutting-edge scientific discussion, the conference had grown to include important opportunities for informal networking and socializing. Participants began to look forward to the annual conference to renew friendships, catch up among colleagues about personal and professional lives, and share personal experiences in their own professional journeys. But the officially designated social time on the conference schedule had become like every other conference: rather stiff, formal, and ill-attended. The WCHEN Research Committee decided to enliven this social time with humor, an exhibition of multiple talents, "a touch of levity" (Benoliel, 1992, p. 127) and much good fun by the invention of an activity unique to any professional gathering. It was named RIFF-RAFF. Joan Shaver, then at the University of Washington, was conscripted to be its leader. Benoliel (1992, p. 127) reported, "RIFF-RAFF was especially important because it allowed us to observe a hidden persona in some our most prestigious and productive investigators."

At the twenty-fifth anniversary of WIN, Shaver submitted a uniquely hilarious must-read account of the beginning of RIFF-RAFF (see Shaver, 1992). Any participant at this and subsequent conferences likely has a personal memory of fierce competition, laughter, embarrassment, or amazement from a RIFF-RAFF performance. According to Shaver (1992, pp. 105-1060), the acronym ostensibly represented "The Regional Institute for Fun and Frivolity (RIFF) . . . [of] The Regional Association of Foremost Flakes" (RAFF). It soon became a highly competitive skit contest among groups represented at WSRN. Winning performances claimed possession of the "Golden D.U.N.G. (Dynamite Ubiquitous Nursing Gumption) Award" (Shaver, 1992, p. 107), to which the winning team would add some token, until it eventually became a rather grotesque, but beloved, addition to the winning institution's trophy case. Following is just a taste of Shaver's delightful story of how it all began (with assumed real identities in brackets):

> . . . This was how to "save" a waning event, "resuscitate" those who gathered at it and otherwise "breathe life" into an obligatory social gathering that had forever occurred at the annual "big meeting of the minds" . . . It was there that Joan . . . suggested that there might be cowpokes on the lazy WSRN who had talents of a different sort, talents that would amaze those who were privileged to experience it. So she begged and pleaded with "Big Daddy" Martin (the leader of the band) [Chair Clair Martin from the University of Alaska], "Tinsel Town" Betty C. [Betty Chang from the University of California Los Angeles], "the Promoter" Annie from little LA on the deserts of AZ [Ann Muhlenkamp

65

from Arizona State University], and Jeanne, Mother Superior [Jeanne Kearns] of the lazy WSRN, among others around the table to arrange a submeeting of the minds (or was it a meeting of the subminds?) perhaps a meeting of small minds. The mousy assistant one from the U-dub [Joan Shaver] argued that this could be a new and wondrous activity at the "big meetings of the minds." But alas, they looked at her vacantly, searching for some sense (or was it dollars?) to this vague and risky scheme. Finally, in desperation, and to avoid conflict (remember that "Big Daddy" was a "shrink" nurse), they granted dispensation and in a magnanimous (or was it obscene?) gesture and with consensus rarely evidenced, chorused, "You do it" (Shaver, 1992, p. 105).

And she did it! Every WSRN member at the time has unforgettable images, such as Lil Likert, Ann Voda's flashing menopause lights (Benoliel, 1992, p. 129), or Carol Ashton's *Beano* apron. Joan Shaver invented and boldly produced a one-of-a-kind feature that promoted enduring friendships and encouraged others to extend themselves in a safe (though surreal) talent-sharing event to complement the significant serious work of *Communicating Nursing Research*.

1984: *Advancing Nursing Science: Qualitative and Quantitative Approaches* - San Francisco, California
Anna Shannon, from Montana State University, was elected Chair of the WCHEN Executive Board, and she was replaced on the program committee by Jean Lum from the University of Hawaii (WIN, 1992, p. 400). The conference of 1984 featured two complementary Keynotes. Jeanne Benoliel, from the University of Washington, spoke on qualitative methods, and Jan Atwood, from the University of Arizona described quantitative approaches.

The WCHEN organization had matured to the point of awarding Emeriti status to some of its pioneers (WIN, 2007, p. 44). The first five members granted such status were members of the original Committee of Seven: Amelia Leino, University of Wyoming; Katherine Hoffman, University of Washington; Kathryn Smith Lasterto, University of Colorado; Lulu Wolf Hassenplug, University of California Los Angeles; and Pearl Coulter, University of Arizona (WIN, 2007, p. 55) (See Appendix H).

The Research Information Exchange
By 1984, graduate programs in nursing had proliferated across the West. To encourage research among graduate students, the "Research Information Exchange" was added to the conference (Rawlinson, 1992). Clair Martin (1992, p. 117) recalled how it worked:

Each member school was permitted to select five of their own master's and five doctoral students to participate in the session . . . The format, a poster session, permitted maximum opportunity for individualized presentations and interaction with interested persons. It was planned to be low key, informal, and supportive. The intent was to enable new scholars to share their research in a non-threatening context and to positively reinforce their efforts so that a pattern of continuing research productivity would be established.

66

The first year, 71 students presented their research. Not only was this successful in the goals for research and professional development, but also increased the number of conference participants to alleviate some budgetary concerns. A new "vitality" was added to the culture and future of the conference (Martin, 1992).

A Second "Committee of Seven"

Also in 1984, a new "Committee of Seven" was appointed by WCHEN to explore the status of the organization and its relationship to WICHE. Behind the scenes, several factors had emerged and combined across time to seriously complicate the relationship between WICHE and WCHEN. The assignment of this new committee was daunting.

Members of the new Committee of Seven represented associate, baccalaureate, and graduate programs in nursing as well as nursing practice (See Note 3-B). Members were Ellamae Branstetter, from Arizona State University; Gerry Hansen, Director of the Nursing Program at Weber State College in Ogden, Utah (one of the first seven associate degree programs in the Mildred Montag's pilot project ["ADN nursing," 2003; Haase, 1990, WSU, 2017; see Note 3-A]); Carol Lindeman, Chair-Elect of WCHEN and Dean of the School of Nursing at Oregon Health and Science University; Jean Lum (Chair of WCHEN and Dean of the School of Nursing at the University of Hawaii at Manoa; Frankie Manning, Chief of Nursing Service at the Veterans Administration Medical Center in Seattle, Washington; Patricia Schmidt, Chair of Nursing Education at Palomar College, San Marcos, California; and Anna Shannon, Dean of the College of Nursing at Montana State University in Bozeman. Executive staff support was provided by Jeanne Kearns ("Report," 1984).

Ellamae Branstetter was described in Chapter 2. She was a presenter at the second *Communicating Nursing Research* conference, enduring critique by the master, Madeleine Leininger (Batey, 1969). She was a member of the conference planning committee in 1973 and Chair of the executive committee that initiated the founding of the Western Society for Research in Nursing. She was indeed among the early pioneers of WCHEN.

Geraldine (Gerry) Hansen was born in Pagosa Springs, Colorado and lived in Oregon and Washington during childhood, but spent most of her life in Ogden, Utah. She was indeed a child of the West. She earned degrees in nursing from Weber State College in Ogden and the University of Utah, and she earned the Ed.D. from Brigham Young University in Provo, Utah. Her entire career was at Weber State University, beginning as an instructor and culminating as Director of the nursing program. She also served on several committees with the National League for Nursing. In addition, she was a Lieutenant Colonel in the U. S. Army Reserves and served in Desert Storm. She died in Ogden at the age of 72 in 2008 (Lindquist, 2008).

Carol Lindeman is described earlier in this chapter. She brought to this Committee of Seven a perspective of the history of the organization, of its mission and activities, and her unique experience of leadership.

Jean Loui Jin Lum was born and reared in Honolulu, Hawaii. She earned the B.S. from the University of Hawaii in 1960, the M.S. from the University of California San Francisco, and the M.A. and Ph.D. from the University of Washington (Honolulu Star-Advertiser, 2016; University of Hawaii, 2001). Her research focused on patient experiences with cancer as well as nursing leadership (see Itano, et al., 1983; Lum, 1970; 1977; 1979; Lum, et al., 1978). She was devoted to WCHEN, and served as Chair of the Research Steering Committee and the committee that initiated the Western Society for Research in Nursing. She died at age 77 in Honolulu in 2015.

Frankie Manning began her career in Tulsa, Oklahoma as a staff nurse specifically designated for African American patients. From her experiences with the National Black Nurses' Association, she established the Wichita Black Nurses Association in Kansas in 1973 (WBNA, 2015). She worked in the United States Army Nurse Corps as head nurse, Director of Quality Improvement, and Chief Nurse and Director of Education. She was deployed to Saudi Arabia, assigned as special assistant to the commander for the 50th General Hospital. She was Chair of WIN in 1989 (WIN, 2016b). She retired in 2000 as Lieutenant Colonel after 22 years of military service. She continues to be active in many public health endeavors in the state of Washington (WSNA, 2012). In 2003, she received the Secretary's Award for Excellence in Nursing from the Department of Veterans Affairs for her work to develop a same day unit, outreach health screening program, continuous care clinic, restraint-free environment, and the position of woman veteran's coordinator (Veterans Affairs, 2003). She was the first nurse to serve on the King County Board of Health and was appointed by the Governor in 2004 to serve on the Washington State Board of Health and later on the Governor's Interagency Council on Health Disparities (WSNA, 2012).

Patricia Schmidt was born in Chicago, Illinois and grew up in the general Chicago area. She earned the B.S. at the College of Saint Teresa in Winona, Minnesota, the M.S. from Marquette University in Milwaukee, and later the Ed.D. from the United States International University in San Diego. She taught in the baccalaureate nursing program at Saint Mary's campus of the Mayo Clinic in Rochester, Minnesota. While there, she drove across country with a roommate to a wedding in San Diego, where she met the man who eventually became her husband, and she moved to California. From 1966 to 1970, she taught nursing at San Diego State University, then spent the remainder of her career as Chair of the Department of Nursing, faculty, and Interim Dean at Palomar College. While there, she was active among the leadership of associate degree programs in the southern California area. She is now emerita faculty at Palomar and continues to live in southern California (Palomar College, 2008; P. Schmidt, personal communication, January 23, 2017).

Anna Shannon is described in Chapter 2. She continues to be a well-known leader in the West and supporter of WIN. She brought to this Committee of Seven her commitment and history with the organization.

The committee convened in Portland, Oregon in October of 1984. With the arrival of Executive Director, Phillip Sirotkin, in 1976, the internal climate of WICHE had changed. Facing severe budget issues, he had threatened to impose fees on nursing organizations to join WCHEN and was taking steps to narrow the focus of the mission of WICHE just as the nursing program was expanding its mission (Abbott, 2004). Sirotkin's words were raw. He reported that WICHE had projected deficit budgets for the previous several years and that the Commissioners expected a balanced budget at their next meeting. He pointed out that even though WCHEN had been highly productive in securing grant funding, the indirect expenses acquired by the organization had not been sufficient to support the program (see Abbott, 2004). He further stated that "the highest priority" were the "reciprocal interstate student exchanges and information sharing [which were the major work of the Medicine and Dentistry programs]. The health programs [including] . . . Nursing . . . [were] in the . . . last priority at WICHE . . . based on the financial situation, funding for the Nursing Program Unit [would] have to be reduced" ("Report," 1984, p. 4). He then criticized several aspects and activities of WCHEN.

Beyond budgetary challenges, three major other issues discussed in the meeting confirmed the imminent departure of WCHEN from WICHE. First, WCHEN had engaged in "actions related to support for the Equal Rights Amendment" (ERA) ("Report, 1984, p. 5). The Amendment had passed in 1972 and needed ratification within seven years from at least 38 states to become law. Among the 15 states who had refused to ratify were three from the West: Arizona, Nevada, and Utah (ERA, 2015). As early as 1975, the WCHEN General Council officially supported the ERA (see WCHEN, 1975). By 1977, the WCHEN Executive Board "implemented the ERA resolution endorsed by the Council in 1975 by passing a motion to hold no WCHEN meetings in states that have not passed the ERA" (see WICHE & WCHEN, 1977, p. 8). This position was revisited and confirmed by the Council as late as 1983 (see WCHEN, 1983, p. 5; see Note 3-C). (Arizona had hosted the *Communicating Nursing Research* conference in 1975 and not again until 1987; Nevada had hosted in 1972 and not again until 2011; and Utah had hosted in 1970 and not again until 1988) (See Note 3-D). By 1985, the position of the organization to support "equal rights for women" was re-affirmed, but without restrictions on meeting locations among the states of the region (WCHEN, 1985a, p. 8; See Note 3-E). Amidst the transition from WCHEN to WIN, this position, or taking any political stance, though not prohibited, was not supported by WICHE officials (see WCHEN, 1985a, p. 2-3).

Second, Sirotkin confirmed that the focus of WICHE's mission was on education, and "cannot promote service involvement" ("Report," p. 5). From the beginning, under Jo Eleanor Elliott and continuing on, the vision of WCHEN was to make a positive difference in clinical practice. Indeed, WCHEN was expanding to include members from clinical agencies with full voting rights.

Finally, WCHEN was broadening its vision and activities to include promotion of graduate education, research development, inclusion of activities related to practice, and engagement in political policy. These activities were noted to be "no longer consistent with the mission of WICHE" ("Report," p. 5), which had narrowed its focus on professional education, especially on student inter-state exchange programs.

Nevertheless, it was well recognized in the session that nursing was emerging as an independent and autonomous discipline with a growing science. The Committee of Seven responded with a strong and visionary statement:

> The members [of the Committee of Seven] indicated a strong need for a regional nursing organization to continue the development of nursing as an academic and practice discipline and to respond to and to effect changes in society, health care delivery, education, the profession, and the role of women. These rapid changes mandate the continuation of a strong regional voice from nursing, and one that emphasizes the partnership of service and education in the larger social-political environment. Although the primary emphasis would be on nursing, a multi-discipline involvement would be essential ("Report," 1984, p. 5).

So the group moved forward with a plan for a change of the relationship of WCHEN with WICHE to become "affiliate" (see "Report," 1984). A transition plan was outlined for resources and leadership. The committee took the courageous action to recommend that WCHEN separate from WICHE by 1987 and form a new, independent organization to "promote service and education as partners in the profession of nursing and furthering its role in health care" (WIN, 2007, p. 44) with interim support and continuing collaboration with WICHE . Thus, the first Committee of Seven "created the organization," and the second Committee of Seven "kept it alive!" (C. A. Lindeman, personal communication, October 24, 2016). All that was left for the organization was to create a new name.

1985: *Influencing the Future of Nursing Research through Power and Politics -* **Seattle, Washington**
Whether by plan or coincidence, the theme and title of the eighteenth conference, on power and politics, were bold statements of the mission of the organization for nurses in the West and well beyond the specific mission of WICHE. Linda Amos, from the University of Utah, boldly began the conference with a message on the theme. Jean Lum was Chair of the WCHEN Executive Board. The conference program committee included Chair Marjorie Habeeb, University of San Francisco; Julie Schorr, University of Nevada, Reno; Marianne Zalar, Stanford University Medical Center, California; Carol Lindeman, Oregon Health and Science University; with Ann Muhlenkamp and Joan Shaver continuing (WIN, 1992, p. 400).

A Bold New Step: The Western Institute of Nursing
A few months before the conference in 1985, the WCHEN Council accepted the recommendation of the new Committee of Seven and expanded its membership to provide a detailed proposal for a new independent regional nursing organization that would include "identifying the purpose, mission, long and short term goals, specific activities, membership, alternative organization structures, and funding options" for the proposed new organization. New members added to the Committee of Seven were Myrna Warnick, Vice President/Patient Care Services, California Hospital in Los Angeles, and Clair Martin, Dean of the College of Nursing and Health Sciences at the University of Alaska in Anchorage (WCHEN, 1986b).

Myrna Warnick was born in the small coal mining town of Sunnyside, Utah. She graduated from Brigham Young University and earned the M.S. from the University of Utah. She held positions in hospital and nursing administration in Salt Lake City, Utah; Los Angeles, California; and Chicago, Illinois. She was known by colleagues as a fierce and wise leader. One example of her public advocacy was hiring the first male nurse on the labor and delivery unit at her hospital (see Japenga, 1985). She ended her career as a member of the faculty at Brigham Young University. She died in 2009 (*Salt Lake Tribune,* 2009).

Clair Martin graduated from the University of Florida. He has been Dean of schools of nursing at the University of Alaska, University of Colorado, and Emory University. (Auchmutey & Gregg, 2005; Hatcher, 2011; UF, 2006). He was also the President of Cumberland University in Lebanon, Tennessee from 1995 to 2000 (Cumberland University, 2017). He served as Chair and member of the WCHEN Research Steering Committee from 1980 to 1984.

By October, a few months after the conference, the Council officially approved a motion to leave WICHE and create the new organization. The WICHE Commission approved the separation. It was time for independence, and Jeanne Kearns was the person to shepherd in the new era. The organization was continuing to grow and mature. The Western Institute of Nursing (WIN) was about to be born (WIN, 2007, p. 44).

References

Abbott, F. C. (2004). *A history of the Western Interstate Commission for Higher Education: The first 40 years.* Boulder, CO: WICHE. See Note 1-D.

ADN nursing celebrates golden anniversary. (2003). *Nursing Education Perspectives, 24(6),* 287.

Ash, J. S., & Weimer, L. A. (1998, April 17). Interview with Carol Lindeman. In *Oregon Health Sciences University (OHSU) history program and oral history project.* Portland, OR: OHSU.

Auchmutey, P., & Gregg, V. (2005). Hearing their voices. In *Emory Nursing.* Retrieved February 10, 2017 from whsc.emory.edu/_pubs/en/2005spring/hearing-voices.html.

Batey, M. V. (Ed.). (1969). *Communicating Nursing Research, 2.* Boulder, CO: WCHEN.

Batey, M. V. (1977). Preface. In M. B. Batey (Ed.), *Communicating Nursing Research, 10* (pp. v-vii). Boulder, CO: WCHEN.

Benoliel, J. Q. (1992). The changing climate of WSRN conferences. In *The anniversary book: A history of nursing in the West 1956-1992* (pp. 125-129). Boulder, CO: WIN.

Brink, P. J. (1992). The *Western Journal of Nursing Research.* In *The anniversary book: A history of nursing in the West 1956-1992* (pp. 57-61). Boulder, CO: WIN.

Culver, V. (2007, April 10). Higher-ed policy guru an energizer. *The Denver Post.* Retrieved September 25, 2016 from http://www.denverpost.com/2007/04/10/higher-ed-policy-guru-an-energizer/.

Cumberland University. (2017). Presidents through history. Retrieved February 10, 2017 from www.cumberland.edu/inauguration/history.

Denver7 (2016, April 11). *7Everyday Hero Jeanne Kearns welcomes visitors to the Denver Art Museum.* Retrieved January 11, 2017 from https://www.youtube.com/watch?v=T5CFYsjfIJg.

Donaldson, S. K., & Crowley, D. M. (1978). The discipline of nursing. *Nursing Outlook, 26(2),* 113-120.

ERA: The Equal Rights Amendment. (2015). Retrieved January 23, 2017 from http://www.equalrightsamendment.org/.

Gaines, B. C. (2000). *Oregon Health Sciences University (OHSU) School of Nursing: A history of the school 1910-1995.* Portland, OR: OHSU.

Gortner, S. R. (1979). Nursing science in transition. In *Communicating Nursing Research, 12* (pp. 121-131). Boulder, CO: WCHEN.

Gortner, S. R. (1992). The federal role. In *The anniversary book: A history of nursing in the West 1956-1992* (pp. 63-67). Boulder, CO: WIN.

Haase, P. T. (1990). *The origins of associate degree nursing.* Durham, NC: Duke University Press.

Hatcher, C. (2011). *All in the timing: From operating room to board room.* Bloomington, IN: Aughorhouse.

Honolulu Star-Advertiser. (2016, January 31). Obituary: Jean Loui Jin Lum. Retrieved January 22, 2017 from http://obits.staradvertiser.com/2016/01/31/jean-loui-jin-lum-2/.

Itano, J., Tanabe, P., Lum, L. J., Lamkin, L., Rizzo, E., Wieland, M., & Sato, P. (1983). Compliance of cancer patients to therapy. *Western Journal of Nursing Research, 5(1),* 5-20.

Japenga, A. (1985, February 17). Not always what doctor ordered: Male nurse Mike Meyer is a minority within a minority. *Los Angeles Times.* Retrieved February 10, 2017 from http://www.articles.latimes.com/1985-02-17/news/vw-3865_1_male-nurse.

Kearns, J. M. (2003). Thank you, Dr. Pamela Brink. *Western Journal of Nursing Research, 25(8)*, 909-910.

King, C. S., & Lindeman, C. A. (1995). The way forward: An interview with Carol Lindeman. Interview by Cheryl Slagle King. *Advanced Practice Nursing Quarterly, 1(1)*, 49-52.

Krueger, J. C. (1992). An historical perspective on nursing research utilization. In *The anniversary book: A history of nursing in the West 1956-1992* (pp. 93-98). Boulder, CO: WIN.

Krueger, J. C., & Nelson, A. H. (1977, March). *Nursing research support and the need for doctorally prepared faculty in educational institutions in the West.* Boulder, CO: WICHE & WCHEN.

Lindeman, C. A. (1974, August). *Delphi survey of clinical nursing research priorities.* Boulder, CO: WICHE & WCHEN.

Lindeman, C. A. (1980). Keynote address: The challenge of nursing research in the 1980s. In *Communicating Nursing Research, 13.* Boulder, CO: WCHEN.

Lindeman, C. A. (1992). Nursing research development. In *The anniversary book: A history of nursing in the West 1956-1992* (pp. 89-92). Boulder, CO: WIN.

Lindquist Mortuary (2008). Geraldine Lattin Hansen. Retrieved January 22, 2017 from http://www.lindquistmortuary.com/notices/Geraldine-Hansen.

Lum, J. L. (1970). Interaction patterns of nursing personnel. *Nursing Research, 19(4)*, 324-330.

Lum, J. L. (1977). Discussion: Symbolic interaction theory as a conceptual foundation for clinical nursing research. *Community Nursing Research, 8,* 345-351.

Lum, J. L. (1979). WICHE panel of expert consultants report: Implications for nursing leaders. *Journal of Nursing Administration, 9(7),* 11-19.

Lum, J. L. J. (1992). Perspective from inside and outside of the organization. In *The anniversary book: A history of nursing in the West 1956-1992* (pp. 123-124). Boulder, CO: WIN.

Lum, J. L., Chase, M., Cole, S. M., Johnson, A., Johnson, J. A., & Link, M. R. (1978). Nursing care of oncology patients receiving chemotherapy. *Nursing Research, 27(6),* 340-346.

Martin, C. E. (1992). The research information exchange for students. In *The anniversary book: A history of nursing in the West 1956-1992* (pp. 115-118). Boulder, CO: WIN.

Midwestern Higher Education Compact (MHEC). (2016). *Phillip L. Sirotkin award: MHEC's highest award.* Retrieved January 21, 2017 from http://www.mhec.org/about-us/phillip-l-sirotkin-award-mhecs-highest-award.

Mitsunaga, B. K. (1992). A turning point in *Communicating Nursing Research.* In *The anniversary book: A history of nursing in the West 1956-1992* (pp. 83-87). Boulder, CO: WIN.

Palomar College. (2008). *Catalogue.* Retrieved January 23, 2017 from http://www2.palomar.edu/pages/catalog/files/2016/05/2008_s9faculty.pdf.

Rawlinson, M. E. (1992). Contributions of posters and symposia to research communication. In *The anniversary book: A history of nursing in the West 1956-1992* (pp. 109-114). Boulder, CO: WIN.

Report of WCHEN's Committee of Seven Meeting. (1984, October 8-9). Document from WIN Archives, Portland, OR.

Salt Lake Tribune. Obituary: Myrna Loy Williams Warnick. Retrieved February 10, 2017 from http://www.legacy.com/obituaries/saltlaketribune/obituary.aspx?pid=134674942.

Shannon, A. M. (1992). WSRN as a society within WIN or WSRN within WCHEN/ WIN: A nested, repeated measures design. In *The anniversary book: A history of nursing in the West 1956-1992* (pp. 133-134). Boulder, CO: WIN.

Shaver, J. (1992). Dances with RiffRaff: The tale of many supertalents. In *The anniversary book: A history of nursing in the West 1956-1992* (pp. 105-108). Boulder, CO: WIN.

University of Florida (UF). (2006). News from the UF College of Nursing. *The Gator Nurse, 2(1).* Retrieved February 10, 2017 from http://ufalumni.ufl.edu/ Newsletters/Nursing/NewsLetter_200608.html.

University of Hawaii at Manoa. (2001). *Catalogue.* Retrieved January 22, 2017 from http://www.catalog.hawaii.edu/00-01/2000html/emeriti-l.htm.

Veterans Affairs. (2003). Secretary's awards for excellence in nursing 2003. Retrieved January 22, 2017 from http://va.gov/opa/pressrel/includes/viewPDF.cmf?id=605.

Ward, M. J. (1992). The compilation of nursing research instruments projects. In *The anniversary book: A history of nursing in the West 1956-1992* (pp. 99-103). Boulder, CO: WIN.

Washington State Nurses Association (WSNA). (2012). Frankie Manning. *WSNA hall of fame.* Retrieved January 22, 2017 from https://www.wsna.org/hall-of-fame/2012/Frankie-Manning/.

Weber State University (WSU). (2017). *History of Weber State School of Nursing.* Retrieved January 12, 2017 from www.weber.edu/Nursing/history.html.

Western Council on Higher Education for Nursing (WCHEN). (1975, October 22-24). Minutes of meetings of the annual WCHEN Council in Seattle, WA. WIN Archives, Portland, OR.

Western Council on Higher Education for Nursing (WCHEN). (1983, February 24-25). Minutes of meetings of the annual WCHEN Council in San Diego, CA. WIN Archives, Portland, OR.

Western Council on Higher Education for Nursing (WCHEN). (1985a, February 20-22). Minutes of meetings of the annual WCHEN Council in San Francisco, CA. WIN Archives, Portland, OR.

Western Council on Higher Education for Nursing (WCHEN). (1985b). Minutes of meetings of the WCHEN Executive board. WIN Archives, Portland, OR.

Western Institute of Nursing (WIN). (1992). *The anniversary book: A history of nursing in the West 1956-1992.* Boulder, CO: WIN.

Western Institute of Nursing (WIN). (2007). *The anniversary book: 50 years of advancing nursing in the West 1957-2007.* Portland, OR: WIN.

Western Institute of Nursing (WIN). (2013). *Communicating Nursing Research, 46; WIN Assembly, 21.* Portland, OR: WIN.

Western Institute of Nursing (WIN). (2014). *Communicating Nursing Research, 47; WIN Assembly 22.* Portland, OR: WIN.

Western Institute of Nursing (WIN). (2015). *The Carol A. Lindeman award for a new researcher.* Retrieved January 19, 2017 from http://www.winursing.org/~mcneilp/ index.php?query=CAROL%20A.%20LINDEMAN.

Western Institute of Nursing (WIN). (2016a). *Communicating Nursing Research, 49.* Portland, OR: WIN.

Western Institute of Nursing (WIN). (2016b). History subcommittee: Potential interviewees for the 50th anniversary project. WIN archives, Portland, OR.

Wichita Black Nurses Association (WBNA). (2015). Association history. *Wichita Black Nurses.* Retrieved January 22, 2017 from http://wichitablacknurses.com/ Options/OurStory.

Notes

3-A. The original seven associate degree programs in the Montag pilot project that began in 1953, funded by the W. K. Kellogg Foundation and following Montag's dissertation, were the following:
Weber State College, Ogden, Utah
Fairleigh Dickinson College, Rutherford, New Jersey
Pasadena City College, Pasadena, California
Henry Ford Community College, Dearborn, Michigan
Orange County Community College, Middletown, New York (Now SUNY Orange)
Virginia Intermont College, Bristol, Virginia
Virginia State College, Norfolk, Virginia

3-B. Documents of the time through much of the early history of WIN use the term "nursing service" to indicate what has become revised in current jargon to be "nursing practice." Herein, the term "practice" is used.

3-C. Minutes of the WCHEN Council Meeting, February 24-25, 1983 in San Diego, CA show the following: "It was moved by Mary Ann Preach and seconded that WCHEN should continue its position of not holding major meetings in those states which did not pass the Equal Rights Amendment passed 34 in favor and 29 against" (p. 5).

3-D. Following is a listing of state locations of *Communicating Nursing Research* conferences:
Arizona
1973, 1975, 1987, 1994, 1998, 2003, 2010
California
1974, 1980, 1984, 1989, 1992, 1995, 1999, 2002, 2005, 2008, 2013, 2016
Colorado
1977, 1979, 1982, 1990, 1996, 2000, 2017
Nevada
1971, 1972, 2011
New Mexico
1981, 1991, 2006, 2015
Oregon
1978, 1983, 1986, 1997, 2004, 2007, 2012
Utah
1968, 1969, 1970, 1988, 2009
Washington
1976, 1985, 1993, 2001, 2014

3-E. In the WCHEN Council Meeting of February 20, 1985 (see WCHEN, 1985), "it was moved by Anna Shannon, seconded by Linda Amos, and unanimously passed to adopt the following resolution:"
WHEREAS the membership of the new western nursing organization affirms its commitment to equal rights for women; and
WHEREAS our previous organization sought to influence equal rights legislation through economic boycott of states which did not take the positive legislation on the Equal Rights Amendment; and
WHEREAS the Equal Rights Amendment legislation is now moot, but equal rights remains a commitment of nursing in the western region; and
WHEREAS the economic boycott method employed did not have its desired effect; Therefore, be it
RESOLVED, that the new organization reaffirm its strong commitment to equal rights for women; and be it

RESOLVED further that the Executive Board be directed to develop a means of making this commitment known without restricting meetings from states in our Western region.

Chapter Four

Communicating Nursing Research, 1986-1999: "BROADENED HORIZONS," "SILVER THREADS," AND THE SCIENCE GROWS

Chapter Four
Communicating Nursing Research, 1986-1999: "BROADENED HORIZONS," "SILVER THREADS," AND THE SCIENCE GROWS

Truly Pearl Coulter's "winds of change" blew again (see Coulter, 1963) and the times reflected Benoliel's "broadened horizons" (Benoliel, 1992, p. 127), as the new western regional organization for nursing became independent of the Western Interstate Commission on Higher Education (WICHE). The first order of business was the selection of a new name. The organizational representatives considered several names, such as "Western Regional Organization for Nursing" (WRON) or "Western Regional Nursing Organization" (WRNO). Jeanne Kearns light-heartedly recalled another name "something like the 'Western Interstate Nursing Organization (WINO)'. Wouldn't that have been great!" (J. Kearns, personal communication, February 1, 2017). The name selected in the end was just right, with the perfect acronym: the Western Institute of Nursing (WIN).

The Western Institute of Nursing
The now independent WIN was organized anew. The commitment of nurses in the West to practice, profession, and society, as well as to education and research was recognized formally in the organization of the Board of Governors, General Assembly, Governing Assembly, and committees established according to its new bylaws, and the provision for societies officially included the Western Society for Research in Nursing (WSRN) (see "Report," p. 5). Jeanne Kearns was the Executive Director (WIN, 1992, p. 15). The mission and goals were adopted (see WIN, 2007, p. 44-45):

The mission of WIN is to influence positively the quality of healthcare for people in the West through monitoring relevant issues and trends and through designing, implementing, and evaluating regional action-oriented nursing strategies in nursing education, nursing practice, and nursing research.

The goals of WIN are to:
1. Promote proactive stances to health care issues and trends which foster the partnership between nursing practice and nursing education;
2. Promote a strong regional voice and network for nursing in the West;
3. Promote quality nursing educational programs that are responsive to the evolving needs of the health care delivery system;
4. Promote quality nursing practice through innovative approaches to the delivery of health care;
5. Facilitate the development of nurse leaders;
6. Monitor and project requirements for nursing in the West, based on societal trends and health care issues;
7. Promote strong regional societies which promote improvement or advancement of nurses and nursing.

Membership with voting privileges was opened to schools of nursing, health care agencies, and individuals in the West. Other types of membership were also included. Under the new organization of WIN, WSRN was the official society to advance the research mission and sponsor the *Communicating Nursing Research* conference that continued to thrive. Benoliel (1992, p. 127) called this period "Broadened Horizons" and recalled the general social climate of subdued economy, the AIDS epidemic, "abortion politics," and increasing engagement in social issues that relate to health care. Such issues were part of the expanded portfolios of research presented at the conference. It was a new dawn for nursing in the West. Research presentations at the Communicating Nursing Research conference reflected the needs, trends, and topics of the American and global society of the time.

Advancing Nursing Research at the Federal Level: Contributions from the West
The history of nursing research in the West was always closely tied to the growth in national attention to research. The story of progress in support for nursing research at the federal level is interesting and bumpy. From the beginning, leaders of WIN enjoyed positive relationships and funding from the Division of Nursing, which had a long history of attention to nursing education, practice, and research. Indeed, the first extramural nursing research program came from the Research Grants and Fellowship Branch of the Division in 1955 (NINR, 2016). The idea of an institute for nursing research at the National Institutes of Health (NIH) was controversial, with leaders both inside and outside the discipline insisting that support for nursing research should remain with the Division and should not be part of NIH. It did not help that President Ronald Reagan opposed it (see Cantelon, 2010; Dumas & Felton, 1984; Gornick & Lewin, 1984; Houser & Player, 2004; Jacox, 2013; See Note 4-1).

Nevertheless, after considerable struggle and controversy, by the end of 1985, federal law authorized the establishment of the National Center for Nursing Research (NCNR) within NIH. Historian Cantelon noted that among the leaders from the West who witnessed and helped to make the history as pathbreakers toward the reality of an institute for nursing research were Kathleen Dracup, Jo Eleanor Elliott, Ada Sue Hinshaw, Patricia Moritz, and Nancy Woods (see Cantelon, 2010). The Center became reality in April 1986, and physician Doris H. Merritt was named acting interim director. She had experience at NIH and been the first woman to chair the Board of Regents at the National Library of Medicine (NLM, 2015). She soon became the mentor for the West's own Ada Sue Hinshaw who became the first Director of the Center (Houser & Player, 2004). Hinshaw led the Center to become the National Institute of Nursing Research (NINR) in 1993 (NINR, 2016).

Ada Sue Hinshaw was born in Arkansas City, Kansas and spent her childhood in the tiny rural town of Cherryvale, Kansas. She graduated from the University of Kansas and earned the M.S. in nursing from Yale University. She then became a faculty member at the University of California San Francisco. Hinshaw was among the five presenters at the first conference in 1968 (see Chapter 2). It was from responses to her presentation at that meeting she decided to move to the University of Arizona for doctoral studies. There she earned the M.S. and Ph.D. in sociology. She became a faculty member at Arizona and clinical researcher at the University of Arizona Medical Center. She helped to build the doctoral program and an impressive research program, for which she gave credit to her team that included Agnes Aamodt, Jan Atwood, Janelle Krueger, Alice Longman, Jesse Peregrin, and Gladys Sorensen (Houser & Player, 2004). The team was always committed to nursing research grounded in clinical practice. In 1985, she was elected Chair of the American Nurses Association Cabinet on Nursing Research, where she joined the cause to establish an institute for nursing research at

NIH. When the NCNR was established and she was offered the position of its director, she was ambivalent at first because of her desire to remain in Arizona where she had family and professional roots. But she accepted and worked to build a foundation for the Institute to happen. In 1989, she hired the West's Carolyn Murdaugh to develop the intramural research program. Hinshaw and her staff worked to lay the foundation for the future (Houser & Player, 2004). In 1992, at her congressional testimony, she gave credit to the Division of Nursing at HRSA for "[training] great nurse researchers [who] had laid a phenomenal foundation for rigorous science" (Houser & Player, 2004, p. 122). By the time of the establishment of the National Institute for Nursing Research (NINR), the budget had grown under Hinshaw's leadership from five million dollars to nearly 50 million dollars (Houser & Player, 2004). Hinshaw later became the Dean of the School of Nursing at the University of Michigan from 1994 to 2006 and the Dean of the Graduate School of Nursing at Uniformed Services University of the Health Sciences in Bethesda, Maryland from 2006 until her retirement in 2014. She was president of the American Academy of Nursing from 1999 to 2001 and received numerous prestigious awards including 13 honorary degrees.

Throughout the history of NINR, leaders from the West have contributed to its success. For example, the following have served or currently serve on the National Advisory Council for Nursing Research of NINR: Dyanne Affonso, Julie Anderson, Patricia Archbold, James Corbett, Marie Cowan, J. Randall Curtis, George Demiris, Glenna Dowling, Kathleen Dracup, Betty Ferrell, Rosanne Harrigan, Felicia Hodge, William Holzemer, Doris Howell, Jillian Inouye, Karin Kirchoff, Deborah Koniak-Griffin, Jean Lum, Courtney Lyder, Bernadette Melnyk, Francis Munet-Vilaro, Carmen Portillo, Kathleen Potempa, Marla Salmon, Mary Siantz, Betty Smith-Williams, Clarann Weinert, Betty Williams, and Nancy Woods (Archive of Council Minutes, 2017; Cantelon, 2010, pp. 241-246; National Advisory Council for Nursing Research, 2017).

1986: *The Winds of Change: New Frontiers in Nursing Research* - Portland, Oregon and
1987: *Collaboration in Nursing Research: Advancing the Science of Human Care* - Tempe, Arizona
Fully in tune with the national movement to embrace and enhance research in nursing, the 1986 conference format and its sessions reflected an increasingly broad range of topics and choices for professional discourse. Carol Lindeman, from Oregon Health and Science University, was Chair of the WCHEN Executive Board and Chair of what was now called the WIN Board of Governors. Program committee members were Chair Marianne Zalar, Stanford University Medical Center, California; Sandra Ferketich, University of California San Francisco; Julie Schorr, University of Nevada, Reno; Marilyn Stember, University of Colorado Health Sciences Center; Virginia Tilden, Oregon Health and Science University; and Marylou McAthie, Sonoma State University, California (WIN, 1992, p. 401). In 1987, Sandra Ferketich became the chair, and new members were Karin Kirchhoff, University of Utah & Hospital; Merle Mishel, University of Arizona; and Elizabeth Nichols, University of Wyoming.

The Keynote Address for 1986 was given by Nancy Woods, who brought history and future together in her speech, "The Winds of Change." In 1987, two Western scholars spoke: Jean Watson on "Academic and Clinical Collaboration: Advancing the Art and Science of Human Caring" and Sue Hegyvary on "Collaboration in Nursing Research:

Advancing the Science of Human Care." The New Researcher Award became officially called the Carol A. Lindeman Award for a New Researcher, in recognition if its founder. Winners were Gwenyth Gerhard from the University of Lowell, Massachusetts and Frederica O'Connor from the University of Washington (WIN, 1986; 1987).

The Research Information Exchange for graduate students (which began in 1984) was expanded to include an additional Research Information Exchange for nurses in clinical practice (Murdaugh, 1992; Rawlinson, 1992). Though nurses in patient care settings had participated in the conference, this new mechanism provided a more formal opportunity to encourage engagement by researchers in clinical practice. Research directly related to patient care had been a continuing value, but was sometimes overshadowed by the focus and sheer number of conference participants from academic settings. By 1987, a few clinical agencies had established nurse researcher positions. These pioneers broke the path for credibility and actual practice of research in the care setting and likely laid the foundation for the future movement that embraced evidence-based practice.

1988: *Nursing: A Socially Responsible Profession* - **Salt Lake City, Utah**
Two important additions became part of the *Communicating Nursing Research* conference in 1988. The first was the Distinguished Research Lectureship, presented, "to [recognize] a senior investigator whose research career has made substantial and sustained contributions to nursing," with the honor going to Ramona Mercer from the University of California San Francisco. (Benoliel, 1992; WIN, 2007, pp. 56-57). This lectureship has continued throughout the history of the conference. The lectures began as reflections on the speaker's career journey in research, including challenges, rewards, and advice. Later, as the science has matured, the focus moved more to scientific reflections on research trajectories related to specific areas of study. The listing of awardees appears as a "who's who" in nursing research not only in the region, but in the country and the world (See Appendix B).

The second addition was the Jo Eleanor Elliott Leadership Award. It was established by Jeanne Kearns to honor Elliott for her outstanding leadership of WCHEN. The first recipient was Anna Shannon of Montana State University. Awardees are nominated by two sponsors, selected by a committee, and recognized for distinguished leadership. As of 2017, 24 leaders have been honored with the award (WIN, 2007, p. 56; See Appendix I). The organization and its research conference were growing toward the future, and at the same time reflecting respect for its history and pioneers with these awards and special designations.

In 1988, the conference also included a special focus session featuring a panel of experts on the AIDS epidemic, a significant health and societal concern at the time (Benoliel, 1992). Judith Saunders of the City of Hope National Medical Center in Duarte, California, was the moderator. Panel members were Anita Eichler of the AIDS Program of the National Institute of Mental Health; Jacqueline H. Flaskerud of the University of California Los Angeles; and Evelyn G. Hartigan of the University of Utah Hospital and College of Nursing.

Anne Davis, of the University of California San Francisco, gave the Keynote Address that affirmed the focus on the responsibility of the profession to society. She explored the concept in the broadest sense, outlining the responsibilities of the profession for specific groups, such as the elderly, the poor, the chronically ill, that health care is a human right, and even advocating against nuclear arms (see Davis, 1988).

Karen Kirchoff of University of Utah and Hospital and University of Utah replaced Sandra Ferketich as Chair of the Program Committee, and new members included Judith Saunders, City of Hope National Medical Center, California; Carolyn Webster-Stratton, University of Washington; Clarann Weinert, Montana State University; and Elizabeth Nichols, University of Wyoming. Toni Sullivan, from the University of Southern California, was Chair of the WIN Board of Governors (WIN, 1992, p. 402).

The Research Exchanges for graduate students and for nurses in clinical practice were combined into one unit. This year, 77 projects were featured from 26 institutions and agencies, including Azusa Pacific University; California State University Bakersfield, Dominguez Hills, Fresno, Long Beach, and Los Angeles; Cedars-Sinai Medical Center; Children's Hospital of Denver; Intercollegiate Center for Nursing Education; Montana State University; Oregon Health and Science University; Tucson Medical Center; University of Alaska; University of Arizona; University of California Davis Medical Center, Irvine Medical Center, Los Angeles, and San Francisco; University of Colorado Health Sciences Center; University of Hawaii; University of New Mexico; University of Utah; University of Washington; University of Wyoming; and Veterans Administration of Prescott, Arizona (WIN, 1988).

The year 1988 marked 20 years from the first *Communicating Nursing Research* Conference. It had grown from 5 podium presentations in the first conference in 1968 to 17 podium, 7 symposia, and 29 posters in the tenth year of 1978; to 62 podium, 5 symposia, 33 posters, and 107 projects in the Research Information Exchange in the twentieth conference of 1988.

1989: *Choices Within Challenges* **- San Diego, California**
The Program Committee of WSRN was changed to be called the Executive Committee of WSRN. Members were Chair Judith Saunders, City of Hope National Medical Center, California; Carolyn Murdaugh, University of Arizona and University Medical Center; Elizabeth Nichols, University of Wyoming; Martha (Marty) Stoner, University of Colorado Health Sciences Center and University Hospital; Carolyn Webster-Stratton, University of Washington; and Clarann Weinert, Montana State University. The Chair of the WIN Board of Governors was Frankie Manning from the Veterans Administration Medical Center in Seattle, Washington (WIN, 1992, p. 402).

Carol Lindeman gave a bold Keynote Address that challenged participants to close the "chasm between the nurse researcher and those in nursing practice" (Elliott, 1992, p. 29; Lindeman, 1989). She outlined the challenges to effective nursing research of the past, present, and future, ending with the following message:

We cannot mandate that the mass of nurses value nursing research any more than we can mandate that the public value it. Both will value it when they can see that it makes a difference. The challenge is making it (research) make a difference (in practice). There are many ways to respond to this challenge. My choice is to promote a conception of the nurse as a scholarly practitioner with the full realization that that means

83

major changes in our educational programs, our work settings, and our scientific endeavors. Although this represents a total upheaval of the current situation, if it doesn't occur, I'm afraid the discipline of nursing will develop in isolation of the profession, and nurses will continue as second class citizens in what is viewed by other professionals and the public as an important but ancillary occupation (Lindeman, 1989, p. 7).

A special session with a panel of experts on the growing issue of underserved populations was added to the 1989 conference (Benoliel, 1992). Judith Saunders, of the City of Hope National Medical Center in California, served as moderator. Speakers included Marjorie A. Muecke from the University of Washington; Linda Phillips, Donna L. Vredevoe, Pamela Shuler, and Mary Woo from University of California Los Angeles; and Anna M. Shannon from Montana State University (WIN, 1989).

The Western Academy of Nurses

In 1989, the Governing Board of WIN discussed options to recognize outstanding members of the organization and how to recruit them to further contribute to its mission. When the idea of a Western Academy of Nurses (WAN) was proposed, the obvious concern was whether it might become perceived as a "lesser" version of the American Academy of Nursing. Memories are that the discussion was intense and concluded in support of the new Academy, with commitment to the highest expectations of those named to the Academy as well as of the work of the group. Criteria for appointment are rigorous, including membership in WIN for at least five years, demonstrated excellence in research, practice, and/or education, and sponsorship by two active members of WIN (WIN, 2016b). New members are inducted during the annual conference, and members of the Academy elect officers and meet at least annually during the conference.

The first members to be inducted in 1990 were Marci Catanzaro from the University of Washington and Anna Shannon and Clarann Weinert from Montana State University. The number of new members inducted each year since then has ranged from one to seven. Membership as of 2017 has grown to 96 distinguished members from 10 Western states and two members who reside outside the region (WIN, 2016c).

The Academy has not disappointed in its contributions to enrich the annual conference. It is more than honorary; it is truly a working group. Since 1994, the Academy has sponsored or presented a special panel session as part of the conference, missing only 2004 and 2005. Known as the "WAN Panels," they have been crafted to address real-world problems and current issues in the discipline, including translation to practice, application of evidence, innovations in education, attention to consumers, entrepreneurial activities in nursing, advanced practice, health disparities, community participatory research, and other issues in practice and policy; and they have always included participants from both academic and clinical setting. (See Appendix E).

1990: *Nursing Research: Transcending the 20th Century* - Denver, Colorado

In 1990, Jo Eleanor Elliott returned to offer the Keynote Address. She confirmed the concerns voiced by Carol Lindeman the previous year regarding the need to bring research closer to practice. She also predicted challenges of the future: national health insurance "of some sort," ethics in health care, increasing demographic diversity, increasing technology, accountability, "short funding" at all levels, and "the call for more interdisciplinary efforts" (Elliott, 1990, p. 6).

The conference continued with a special session that featured an expert panel on the growing health issue of substance abuse, continuing the movement toward promoting the responsibility of nurse researchers toward important social issues (Benoliel, 1992; WIN, 1990). The session on substance abuse was moderated by Marylou McAthie, from Sonoma State University in California; and speakers included Mary Haack, Guest Researcher at the National Institutes of Health; Donna Jensen, from Oregon Health and Science University; Juanita Murphy, from Arizona State University; Constance Connell, from the Arizona Board of Nursing; and Elizabeth Pace, Executive Director of N.U.R.S.E.S. of Colorado Corporation (WIN, 1990). Peggy Chinn, from the University of Utah gave a special closing address. She outlined challenges of ethics, praxis, and nursing scholarship for the 21st century (Chinn, 1990).

Elizabeth Nichols, from the University of Wyoming, was Chair of the WIN Board of Governors. The WSRN Program Committee was chaired by Martha "Marty" Stoner, University of Colorado Health Sciences Center and University Hospital, with members Marie Berger, Oregon Health and Science University; Linda Faber, University of California Los Angeles Medical Center; Carolyn Murdaugh, University of Arizona and University Medical Center; Juanita Murphy, Arizona State University; and Elaine Sorensen (Marshall), Brigham Young University (WIN, 1992, p. 403).

1991: *Partnerships: Putting It All Together* - Albuquerque, New Mexico
The year 1991 marked the first combined WIN Assembly (its fifth annual meeting) and WSRN *Communicating Nursing Research* conference (its 24th annual meeting) (WIN, 1992, p. 15). Doris Kearns Goodwin, Pulitzer Prize winning historian, gave the WIN Assembly Keynote, "A Look at the Private Lives of Our Public Figures." A WIN panel addressed "Implementing Recommendations from the Secretary's Commission on Nursing: Leaders in the West Respond." Kathleen Long from Montana State University was moderator, and panelists were Zina Herbert, of Health and Community Services at the Tacoma Lutheran Home and Retirement Center in Washington; Judith Kiernan, of University of Utah Hospital; Cathy Michaels, of Carondelet St Mary's Hospital and Health Center in Arizona; and Jane Scharff, from St. Vincent's Hospital and Health Center in Montana. These were followed by WIN podium sessions (WIN, 1991b).

The Distinguished Research Lecture was given by Patricia Archbold from Oregon Health and Science University. She outlined "An Interdisciplinary Approach to Family Caregiving Research." The Carol Lindeman Award for a New Researcher went to Diana Wilkie, from the University of Washington, for her work on pain coping strategies in patients with lung cancer (WIN, 1991a).

The WIN Assembly featured 12 podium presentations in a meeting that preceded the WSRN research meetings. At the WSRN meeting, a total of 125 research papers were presented (Mitsunaga, 1992, p. 84). Linda Faber took the helm as Chair of the Program Committee with continuing members Marie Berger, Juanita Murphy, and Elaine Sorensen (Marshall), with new members Ginette Pepper, Swedish Medical Center, Colorado, and Virginia Tilden, Oregon Health and Science University (WIN, 1992, p. 403).

Listed on the WSRN program was Keynote Jane Norbeck, from the University of California, on "The Merging of Agendas for Education, Research, and Practice." Her message outlined the history of the profession of nursing from a developmental perspective: "Separate agendas are part of a developmental phase in the history of a profession in which specific elements must be mastered before integration can occur" (Norbeck, 1991a, p. 3). She then challenged the audience to design future models to advance the effective integration of nursing education, research, and practice.

1992: *Silver Threads: 25 Years of Nursing Excellence* - **San Diego, California**
The meeting in 1992 marked 25 years, the silver anniversary, of the *Communicating Nursing Research* conference. The theme, "Silver Threads," was apt, reflecting the lyrics of the old song, "silver threads among the gold." The silver anniversary of a highly successful nursing research conference was nested within the regional organization of WIN, which was truly "golden" in its bold vision and accomplishments. It was a significant time, as the conference was held along with the Sixth Annual WIN Assembly as well as the 35th anniversary of the entire western regional organization (WIN, 2007, p. 46). The speakers were among the best in the discipline.

In 25 years, the conference not only had grown in number and diversity of presentations, but had matured in offerings that promoted analysis, application to practice and policy, and consideration of trajectories and consequences of research in nursing. Carol Lindeman returned with the Keynote Address on "The New Scholarship," and Ada Sue Hinshaw, the Director of the NCNR, delivered a plenary address on "The Impact of Nursing Science on Health Policy." State of the Art presentations included the following: "If Not Now, Then When: Nursing's Research Utilization Imperative" by Nancy Donaldson of the University of California Irvine Medical Center, "Measurement: A Foundation of Nursing Science" by William Holzemer of the University of California San Francisco, "Nursing Research Serving the Underserved: Homeless Health Care" by Ada Lindsey of the University of California Los Angeles, and "Attending to Many Voices: Beyond the Qualitative-Quantitative Dialectic" by Phyllis Schultz of the University of Washington.

Those presentations were followed by round table discussions on additional State of the Art papers by some of the finest researchers in the West, including Ethics Research by Kathleen Chafey, Children's Health by Nancy Hester, Health Promotion Research by Shirley Laffrey, Organizational and Administrative Research by Ruth Ludemann, Cultural Diversity Research by Afaf Meleis, Mental Health Research by Helen Nakagawa-Kogan, Physiological Research by Patsy Perry, Gerontological Research by Linda Phillips, and Women's Health Research by Nancy Woods (WIN, 1992).

The first conference in 1968 featured five papers to an audience of 44 people from the West. Twenty-five years later, over 125 papers were presented to nearly 350 people from across the United States as well as from Canada, Sweden, Samoa, and China (McNeil & Lindeman, in press).

On this occasion, always with an eye on improvement regarding the state of the science and practice in nursing research, Jo Eleanor Elliott (1992, p. 29) warned:

Esoterica of research topics and self-aggrandizement of nurse researchers are issues nursing needs to address head-on. Honesty in nursing science must be a *sine qua non* of all nursing research. The need continues to translate research-generated knowledge to nursing practice and to test practice generated knowledge through research.

Also, looking toward the future by preserving the past, Executive Director Jeanne Kearns and the Program Committee invited pioneers of the past 25 years to write individual eye-witness accounts of the history of WIN, WSRN, and the conference. These were compiled into *The Anniversary Book*. That volume offers a treasury of first-hand, primary sources for this history (see WIN, 1992). Thelma Cleveland, from the Intercollegiate Center for Nursing Education in Washington, was Chair of the WIN Board of Governors. The silver anniversary Program Committee included Chair Virginia Tilden, Oregon Health and Science University; Elizabeth Nichols, University of Wyoming; Adeline Nyamathi, University of California Los Angeles; Ginette Pepper, Swedish Medical Center, Colorado; Patsy Perry, Arizona State University; and Maryann Pranulis, Veterans Administration Medical Center, Utah (WIN, 1992, p. 404).

1993: *Scholarship in Practice* – Bellevue, Washington

In 1993, the WIN Assembly again met with WSRN as part of the *Communicating Nursing Research* conference with proceedings of both meetings in the same volume, though still in separate sections (see WIN, 1993). The WIN Assembly featured Sanford S. Levy, Associate Professor of History and Philosophy at Montana State University as the Keynote speaker on "Moral Theory and Moral Practice: A Philosopher's Perspective." WIN Panels included "Enriching Nursing Education: Applying and Integrating Research Findings" and "Models for Collaboration: Practice, Education, and Research." Eleven podium presentations fell under themes of "Models and Issues for Research in Practice," "Nursing Research: Creating and Solving Nursing Administration Problems," and "Research Utilization in Diverse Settings" (WIN, 1993).

The WSRN Keynote speaker was Sue Hegyvary from the University of Washington, on "Scholarship for Practice in a Changing World" (WIN, 1993). State of the Art and Science Papers included "State of the Art in Quality of Life Research" by Geraldine Padilla, from the University of California Los Angeles, and "Cardiovascular Disease in Women: State of the Science" by Carolyn Murdaugh from the National Center for Nursing Research at NIH. Nancy Woods, of the University of Washington, gave the Distinguished Research Lecture on "Women's Lives, Women's Health." Podium and symposia papers totaled 163 presentations, and twenty-one posters were featured (WIN, 1993).

Kathleen Long, from Montana State University and Jeanne Kearns established the Anna M. Shannon Mentorship Award to "recognize Shannon [Dean Emerita of Montana State University College of Nursing] for her unselfish efforts to support and promote the professional growth of other nurses in the West." The first award went to Phyllis Ethridge of Carondelet St. Mary's Hospital in Tucson, Arizona. By 2017, twenty-seven Shannon Mentorship Awards have been bestowed (see Appendix G).

Ellen Lewis, from the University of California Irvine was Chair of the WIN Board of Governors. Patsy Perry of Arizona State University chaired the conference, with committee members Carrie Jo Braden, University of Arizona; Maureen Keefe, University of Colorado Health Sciences Center; Adeline Nyamathi, University of California Los Angeles, Maryann Pranulis, Salt Lake City VA Medical Center, Utah; and Kay Hart, LDS Hospital, Utah (WIN, 2007, p. 77).

1994: *Research, Practice, and Education Within the Health Care Agenda* – Phoenix, Arizona and
1995: *Innovation and Collaboration: Responses to Health Care Needs* – San Diego, California
In 1994, the first panel presentation by the Western Academy of Nurses appeared on the program. It was titled "Commitment to Advancing Nursing," with topics of "Relationship between WAN and the WIN Mission and Goals and Paradigms of Change" by Clarann Weinert, "Integrating Scholarship into Advanced Practice" by Marci Catanzaro, "Integrating Scholarship into Administration" by Barbara Trehearne, and "Facilitating Faculty Research/Scholarship in a Low Resource Environment" by Chiyoko Furukawa and Janelle Krueger (WIN, 1994). In 1995, the WAN Panel was themed "Collaboration: Innovations for Consumers—Education, Practice, and Research. Speakers included Heather Young on "Collaboration with Consumers," Marie Driever on "Focus on Interdisciplinary Teamwork: A New Form of Collaboration?", Mary Ann Johnson on "Collaboration within Education," and Pamela Baj on "Effective Models of Research Collaboration" (WIN, 1995).

Major speakers addressed issues in health care and nursing of the times. Conferences and speeches also reflected a trend to explicitly list the following three words: "research, practice, and education" within titles. The 1994 and 1995 Keynote speakers were Anne Bavier and Janet Rodgers, respectively. They introduced both WIN and WSRN sessions, as continued into the future, beginning the gradual blending of the sections. State of the Science Papers also addressed topics of growing interest: informatics by Suzanne Henry; rural nursing by Clarann Weinert (WIN, 1994); clinical outcomes research by Patricia Moritz; and research in distance education by Dianna Shomaker (WIN, 1995).

In 1994, Kathleen Long, from Montana State University, was Chair of the WIN Board of Governors. Maureen Keefe moved to chair the WSRN Executive Committee with continuing members Carrie Jo Braden and Kay Hart. New members were William Holzemer, University of California San Francisco, Julie Johnson, University of Nevada, Reno; and Karen Schepp, University of Washington (WIN, 2007, p. 78). By 1995, Michael Rice, from the Intercollegiate Center for Nursing Education in Washington, was Chair of the WIN Board of Governors. Julie Johnson chaired the 28th conference with continuing committee members Carrie Jo Braden, William Holzemer, and Karen Schepp. Elizabeth Nichols of the University of Wyoming rejoined the committee with new member Pamela Baj of San Francisco State University (WIN, 2007, p. 78).

Members of the discipline throughout the country continued to recognize the conference as a model. At the conference in 1995, WIN/WSRN were awarded the 1994-1995 Regional Research Dissemination Award from Sigma Theta Tau International Honor Society for Nursing (WIN, 1995, p. 373; WIN, 2007, p. 46). Also by 1995, several other significant WIN and WSRN honors were added to the program, including naming of WIN Emeriti (this year honorees included Doris Bloch, Beverly McCord, and Verle Waters). The new Anna M. Shannon Mentorship Award went to Ann Voda and Helen Nakagawa-Kogan. Gerry Hansen, of Weber State University, received the Jo Eleanor Elliott Leadership Award; the Carol A. Lindeman Award for a New Researcher went to Patricia Carney; and Joyce Verran gave the Distinguished Research Lecture (WIN, 1995, p. 371) (See Appendices B, C. G, H, I).

1996: *Advancing Nursing through Research, Practice, and Education* – Denver, Colorado
The year 1996 was a poignant time, and fittingly the conference was in Colorado, the home headquarters of WIN/WSRN. Denver was also the home of Jeanne Kearns, who had served the organization for a total of 21 years, and who now announced her retirement. Juanita Tate, from the University of Colorado Health Science Center, gave the Keynote Address on "Advancing Nursing in Turbulent Times: Implications for Practice, Education, and Research," and the panel of the Western Academy of Nurses followed a theme of entrepreneur ventures and innovations in health care (1996). Also in 1996, The Glaxo Wellcome Research Award was presented for the first time, going to Rebecca Dahl, Research Specialist, Community Nursing Organization, Carondelet Health Care Network, Tucson, Arizona.

The Board of Governors decided that it was the right time for WIN to move from the facilities in Boulder, Colorado that it had shared with WICHE. The Board sought proposals for arrangements to host the organization. Following extensive review of proposals from several organizations, the decision was made to move the headquarters of WIN and WSRN to Portland to be housed within Oregon Health and Science University School of Nursing, effective July 1, 1996 (WIN, 2007, p. 46; WIN, 2016). Paula McNeil was appointed Executive Director. WIN leaders involved in the transition report some anxiety and sleepless nights. The challenges of the decision to move, the logistics of the move, the risks in upsetting tradition, and scarce resources to make the move were almost overwhelming. But true to their pioneer heritage in WIN, they eventually achieved success, and the new headquarters in Portland were open for business with significant support from the School of Nursing at Oregon Health and Science University.

A New Executive Director: Paula A. McNeil
Paula A. Paolo McNeil was born in McMinnville, Oregon and raised in the nearby small, rural community of Yamhill, Oregon. She was preparing to enroll in a hospital diploma program in Portland, Oregon until an aunt who was a nurse told her the baccalaureate degree was "the future of nursing". She then enrolled in the University of Oregon (UO) and graduated with a BSN from its Portland campus. Later, she earned a Master's degree with an emphasis in nursing administration from the Oregon Health Sciences University (formerly UO and now OHSU). After her undergraduate education, she was employed as a medical-surgical nurse in Portland and Maui, Hawaii before returning to Oregon to join the staff of the Oregon Nurses Association as the Assistant Executive Director. Within a year, she was promoted to Associate Executive Director and became the Director of Government Relations. She was the first full-time paid lobbyist for ONA, a position she held for a decade before becoming Executive Director. While serving as lobbyist, the 1973 revision of the nurse practice act was enacted in law. Noteworthy in that legislation was the first inclusion of language authorizing advanced practice in Oregon. Subsequently, she served as Executive Director of Oregon Health Decisions, a grassroots, values-based organization that supplied the values of Oregonians used to craft the Oregon Health Plan. McNeil currently serves as both the Executive Director of WIN and assistant professor in the School of Nursing at OHSU (OHSU, 2017).

Ever forward-looking, the last Governing Assembly held before the move to Portland produced amendments to the WIN/WSRN bylaws to merge societies into the central functions of WIN. Functionally and realistically, WSRN has always functioned under WIN, as Shannon had articulated earlier (see Shannon, 1992, pp. 133-134) and the program was structured to integrate the WIN Assembly and WSRN research presentations, though separate program committees continued. Vivian Gedaly-Duff of Oregon Health and Science University, Patsy Perry from Arizona State University, and Nancy White of the University of Northern Colorado joined the Executive Committee of WSRN. Barbara derwinski-Robinson, from Montana State University, was Chair of the WIN Board of Governors (WIN, 1996; WIN, 2007, p. 79).

Paula McNeil was just right to lead WIN in its new location in Oregon. She had the preparation and extensive experience in both non-profit organizations and the new home. Challenges were evident from the beginning of her tenure. WIN was projected to arrive at OHSU with $28,000, but after all the obligations were paid in Colorado, $8,000 was forwarded to the new location. The aforementioned Bylaws amendments resulted in some residual concern about the future direction of the organization, especially the dissolution of WSRN. She undertook those challenges and has led the organization for the last 21 years, effectively managing unprecedented growth of WIN and the *Communicating Nursing Research* conference. She has been creative in use of resources to support such growth, including the assurance that WIN is committed to the *Communicating Nursing Research* conference and the establishment of a reserve fund, sufficient to assure the continuation of WIN, regardless of any economic downturn. Under her leadership, most external funding has been secured to build coalitions and extend educational services among educational institutions and clinical agencies across the entire country. She has presented and published with other WIN members on the current and successful NEXus initiative described in Chapter 5. She was a charter member of Beta Psi Chapter of Sigma Theta Tau International, is a member of the Board of Directors of Oregon Health Decisions, and is a member of the American Society of Association Executives and the Oregon Society of Association Management. Her most recent success has been the leadership of the celebration of the 50th *Communicating Nursing Research* conference.

The Last Three Conferences of the Twentieth Century:
1997: *Nursing: Changing the Environment* – **Portland, Oregon and**
1998: *Quality Research for Quality Practice* – **Phoenix, Arizona and**
1999: *Nursing Research: For the Health of Our Nation* – **San Diego, California**
For unknown reasons, participation in the last three conferences of the twentieth century appeared to level a bit. As noted, ten years earlier in 1988, there were 62 podium, 5 symposia, and 33 posters. The average numbers of the 1997 through 1999 were 53 podium, 9 symposia, 32 posters, and 52 Research Information Exchange projects. Nevertheless, total attendance continued to grow each year.

From 1997 to 1998, Patsy Perry, from Arizona State University, was Chair of the Board of Governors. In 1999, Marie Miller, from the Colorado Area Health Education Center (AHEC) System, became Chair. Officers of the conference program committee during these years were Chairs Nancy White and Marie Driver. Committee members were Carrie Jo Braden, Mary Cadogan, Kathleen (Kay) Chafey, Tina DeLapp, Marie Driever, Vivian Gedaly-Duff, Rose Gerber, Jane Hirsch, Julie Johnson, Martha Lentz, Pamela Mitchell, and Patsy Perry (See WIN, 1997, pp. 79-80; 1998; 1999). In 1998, Paula McNeil led WIN to become incorporated under the nonprofit corporation laws of the state of Oregon (WIN, 2016a).

The volumes of the conference proceedings now showed the two sections of the conference (*WIN Assembly* and *Communicating Nursing Research*) to be increasingly integrated into one program. Symposia were growing in number as were multiple-authored papers, reflecting the maturing of the science to feature a growing focus on research trajectories rather than individual isolated studies. Keynotes for those years included: 1997 - Sue T. Hegevary, University of Washington, on "Nursing: Changing the Environment;" 1998 - Barbara Durand, Arizona State University, on "Quality Research for Quality Practice," and 1999 - Mary Ann Curry, Oregon Health and Science University, on "Strategy and Serendipity: Using Research to Influence Health Policy"—all reflecting issues of the time: continuing the focus on practice and a growing attention to policy (See WIN, 1997; 1998; 1999).

State of the Science papers reflected important trajectories in moving the science of nursing forward on significant contemporary issues in health care. They were by Christine Kasper, from the University of California Los Angeles, on "Skeletal Muscle Atrophy and Fatigue;" Christine Tanner, from Oregon Health and Science University, on "Clinical Judgment and Evidence-Based Practice: Conclusions and Controversies;" Virginia Tilden, from Oregon Health and Science University, on "Dying in America: Ethics and End-of-Life Care;" Gerri Lamb, from Carondolet Health Care in Tucson, Arizona; and Carol Landis, from the University of Washington, on "Current Perspectives in Psychoneuroimmunology for Nursing Research."

The Western Academy of Nurses continued the tradition of boldly addressing current issues always with a view toward the future. In 1997, the WAN panel explored changing contexts and paradigm shifts for practice from a chaos theory perspective. Speakers were Maryann Pranulis, Carol Ashton, Dianna Shomaker, and Marie Driever (WIN, 1997). In 1998, Marci Catanzaro and Mary Ann Johnson formally debated the question, "Should every nurse be a nurse practitioner?" (WIN, 1998). And in 1999, the WAN panel confronted the current sacred cow of evidence-based practice with "Evidence-Based Practice – OR – 'Cookbook' Nursing?" Brave speakers were Christine Tanner, Marie Driever, Patricia Moritz, and Sheila Wheeler (WIN, 1999).

The Science Grows: Contributing to the Advancing Discipline
Since the beginning of WCHEN (now WIN) in 1957, the importance of a vibrant organization to support nursing and nurses in the Western region continued to grow. But the influence of the annual *Communicating Nursing Research* conference, now integrated with the annual *WIN Assembly* meeting, had expanded far beyond its 13 western states. The work of nurses in the West not only reflected a growing national profession, but contributed to the progress and maturity of the science and discipline. Keynote speakers, Distinguished Research Lecturers, State of the Science presenters, WAN panelists, and dozens of podium and symposia presentations were not only leaders in the West, but were nationally recognized scholars and practitioners.

Significant contributions to nursing science continue to come from the scholars of the West. A sample listing of areas of study will call to mind the names of outstanding researchers who presented at the dawn of their careers, who attracted significant funding, who developed the theories, knowledge, and interventions for health improvement, and who continue to mentor new scientists. Just a few areas advanced by researchers of the West are Population Health (Rural, Families, Women, Health Disparities, Ethnically Diverse Communities), Symptom Management (Pain, Chronic

Conditions, Sleep), Biobehavioral Issues, Concepts for Health (Transcendence, Uncertainty), Specific Disease and Health Conditions (HIV/AIDS, Cardiovascular Disease, Cancer), Innovative Methods, Physiologic Phenomena, Nursing Education, Nursing Systems and Health Care Administration. The *Communicating Nursing Research* conference has provided a forum for inspiration, dissemination, critique and review, building teams by networking, discussion and debate, identifying funding resources, and just plain joy in the company of colleagues who share a common interest in making life better for others.

When the *Communicating Nursing Research* conferences began, with few exceptions, "there was neither nurse scientist nor nursing science" (personal communication, M. Batey, February 8, 2017). Early nurses in the West recognized the need for research, even when few were either doing it or prepared to do it. Though they sought mentors and consultants from other disciplines, who often discouraged even the thought of research in nursing, they persisted, worked together to promote graduate education and development of research skills. After the organization of WCHEN, they began immediately to plan for a conference for dissemination, development, and debate—and it continues.

References

Archive of Council Minutes (2011, January 1-19). *National Advisory Council for Nursing Research.* Bethesda, MD: NINR. Retrieved February 7, 2017 from https://www.ninr.nih.gov/aboutninr/nacnr/councilminutesarchive.

Benoliel, J. Q. (1992). The changing climate of WSRN conferences. In *The anniversary book: A history of nursing in the West 1956-1992* (pp. 125-129). Boulder, CO: WIN.

Cantelon, P. L. (2010). *NINR: Bringing science to life.* Bethesda, MD: NINR.

Chinn, P. L. (1990). Toward the 21st century: Nursing theory, research, and practice. In *Communicating Nursing Research, 23* (p. 33). Boulder, CO: WIN.

Coulter, P. P. (1963, July). *The winds of change: Progress report of regional cooperation in collegiate nursing education in the West.* Boulder, CO: WICHE. WIN archives, Portland, OR.

Davis, A. J. (1988). Nursing: A socially responsible profession. In *Communicating Nursing Research, 21* (pp. 1-13). Boulder, CO: WIN.

Dumas, R G., & Felton, G. (1984). Should there be a National Institute for Nursing? *Nursing Outlook, 21(1),* 16-22.

Elliott, J. E. (1992). The West's regional efforts in nursing research. In *The anniversary book: A history of nursing in the West 1956-1992* (pp. 25-30). Boulder, CO: WIN.

Gornick, J. C., & Lewin, L. S. (1984, September 7). *Assessment of the organizational locus of the Public Health Service nursing research activities.* Contract number 282-83-0072, NINR Archives, Box 11. Cited by Cantelon, P. L. (2010). *NINR: Bringing science to life* (pp. 29-310. Bethesda, MD: NINR.

Houser, B., & Player, K. (2004). Chapter 6: Ada Sue Hinshaw. In *Pivotal moments in nursing, volume 1: Leaders who changed the path of a profession* (pp. 105-127). Indianapolis, IN: Sigma Theta Tau International.

Jacox, A. (2013). Response to 60th anniversary issue of *Nursing Outlook, Nursing Outlook,* 61(3), 127-128.

Lindeman, C. A. (1989). Choices within challenges. In *Communicating Nursing Research, 22* (pp. 1-7). Boulder, CO: WIN.

McNeil, P. A., & Lindeman, C. A. (in press). A history of the Western Institute of Nursing and its Communicating Nursing Research conference. *Nursing Research.*

Mitsunaga, B. K. (1992). A turning point in *Communicating Nursing Research.* In *The anniversary book: A history of nursing in the West 1956-1992* (pp. 83-87). Boulder, CO: WIN.

Murdaugh, C. (1992). Research information exchange for clinical agency staff. In *The anniversary book: A history of nursing in the West 1956-1992* (pp. 119-122). Boulder, CO: WIN.

National Advisory Council for Nursing Research (2017). Recent and upcoming Council meetings. Retrieved February 7, 2017 from https://www.ninr.nih.gov/aboutninr/nacnr.

National Institute of Nursing Research (NINR). (2016). History: Important events in the National Institute of Nursing Research history. Retrieved February 4, 2017 from https://www.ninr.nih.gov/aboutninr/history.

National Library of Medicine (NLM). (2015, June 3). Changing the face of medicine. Biography: Dr. Doris Honig Merritt. Retrieved February 4, 2017 from https://cfmedicine.nlm.nih.gov/physicians/biography_224.html.

Norbeck, J. S. (1991). The merging of agendas for education, research, and practice. In *Communicating Nursing Research, 24* (pp. 3-14). Boulder, CO: WIN.

Oregon Health & Science University (OHSU). (2017). Paula A. McNeil. Retrieved February 28, 2017 from http://www.ohsu.edu/xd/education/schools/school-of-nursing/faculty-staff/mcneil-paula-faculty-pg.cfm.

Rawlinson, M. E. (1992). Contributions of posters and symposia to research communication. In *The anniversary book: A history of nursing in the West 1956-1992* (pp. 109-114). Boulder, CO: WIN.

Report of WCHEN's Committee of Seven Meeting. (1984, October 8-9). Document from WIN Archives, Portland, OR.

Shannon, A. M. (1992). WSRN as a society within WIN or WSRN within WCHEN/ WIN: A nested, repeated measures design. In *The anniversary book: A history of nursing in the West 1956-1992* (pp. 133-134). Boulder, CO: WIN.

Tanner, C. A. (1998). Clinical judgement and evidence-based practice: Conclusions and controversies. In *Communicating Nursing Research, 31* (pp. 19-35). Portland, OR: WIN.

Western Council on Higher Education for Nursing (WCHEN). (1986). *Communicating Nursing Research, 19.* Boulder, CO: WICHE/WCHEN.

Western Institute of Nursing (WIN). (1987). *Communicating Nursing Research, 20.* Boulder, CO: WIN.

Western Institute of Nursing (WIN). (1988). *Communicating Nursing Research, 21.* Boulder, CO: WIN.

Western Institute of Nursing (WIN). (1989). *Communicating Nursing Research, 22.* Boulder, CO: WIN.

Western Institute of Nursing (WIN). (1990). *Communicating Nursing Research, 23.* Boulder, CO: WIN.

Western Institute of Nursing (WIN). (1991a). *Communicating Nursing Research, 24.* Boulder, CO: WIN.

Western Institute of Nursing (WIN). (1991b, May 1-4). Fifth Annual WIN Assembly and 24th Annual Communicating Nursing Research Conference Program. WIN Archives, Portland, OR.

Western Institute of Nursing (WIN). (1992). *The anniversary book: A history of nursing in the West 1956-1992.* Boulder, CO: WIN.

Western Institute of Nursing (WIN). (1993). *Communicating Nursing Research, 26; WIN Assembly 1.* Boulder, CO: WIN.

Western Institute of Nursing (WIN). (1994). *Communicating Nursing Research, 27; WIN Assembly, 2.* Boulder, CO: WIN.

Western Institute of Nursing (WIN). (1995). *Communicating Nursing Research, 28; WIN Assembly, 3.* Boulder, CO: WIN.

Western Institute of Nursing (WIN). (1996). *Communicating Nursing Research, 29; WIN Assembly, 4.* Boulder, CO: WIN.

Western Institute of Nursing (WIN). (1997). *Communicating Nursing Research, 30; WIN Assembly, 5.* Portland, OR: WIN.

Western Institute of Nursing (WIN). (1998). *Communicating Nursing Research, 31; WIN Assembly, 6.* Portland, OR: WIN.

Western Institute of Nursing (WIN). (1999). *Communicating Nursing Research, 32; WIN Assembly, 7.* Portland, OR: WIN.

Western Institute of Nursing (WIN). (2007). *The anniversary book: 50 years of advancing nursing in the West 1957-2007.* Portland, OR: WIN.

Western Institute of Nursing (WIN). (2016a). About WIN: History of WIN. Retrieved January 22, 2017 from https://www.winursing.org/about-win/.

Western Institute of Nursing (WIN). (2016b). *Western Academy of Nurses (WAN).* Portland, OR: WIN. Retrieved January 20, 2017 from https://www.winursing.org/western-academy-of-nurses-2/.

Western Institute of Nursing (WIN). (2016c). *WAN Inductees.* Portland, OR: WIN. Retrieved January 20, 2017 from https://www.winursing.org/western-academy-of-nurses-2/western-academy-of-nurses/.

Notes

4-1. The Division of Nursing was part of the Health Resources and Services Administration (HRSA), and its mission became more aligned with the mission of HRSA: "clinical training in the health care professions" (NINR, 2016).

Chapter Five

Communicating Nursing Research, 2000-2017: NATIONAL AND INTERNATIONAL LEGACY AND INFLUENCE

Chapter Five
Communicating Nursing Research, 2000-2017:
NATIONAL AND INTERNATIONAL LEGACY
AND INFLUENCE

By the arrival of the twenty-first century, it was clear that the *Communicating Nursing Research* conference had exceeded the expectations of its early pioneers. The maturity and sophistication of the research and the researchers, as well as the development of nursing science had grown rapidly. The first decade of the new century reflected expansion of the *Communicating Nursing Research* conference in a variety of ways. Numbers of participants, awards, and mechanisms for research development and dissemination, and diversity of topics and presenters continued to grow. Through the 1990s, names of presenters revealed a sharp increase in the number of men and members of ethnic minorities.

Building on the national influence of the organization, representatives from the Western Institute of Nursing (WIN) collaborated with other regional research organizations and the American Academy of Nursing to establish the Council for the Advancement of Nursing Science. This idea developed after the American Nurses Association had restructured and disbanded its Council of Nursing Research.

The goals of the Council are to be a strong voice for nursing science at national and international levels by developing, conducting, and utilizing nursing science, to disseminate research findings across individuals and groups in scientific and lay communities, and to facilitate life-long learning opportunities for nurse scientists (CANS, 2016).

Nationally, the new century was also marked by a series of reports from the Institute of Medicine that directly affected how nursing contributes to health care in the country, including the first report specifically for nursing (see IOM, 2000; 2001; 2003; 2006; 2011). Themes of the conferences reflected conversations and movements in nursing and health care at the national level: innovation, quality, and policy.

The Conference began the 2000s by returning to its place of origin, Colorado. Ironically, this history began in Colorado, this chapter begins in Colorado, and the history and chapter end with the 2017 meetings also in Denver.

2000: *Building on a Legacy of Excellence in Nursing Research* – **Denver, Colorado**
The conference began the new millennium with 100 papers, including 49 podium presentations, 10 symposia, 44 posters, and 37 projects in the Research Information Exchange. It was also the year of the tenth anniversary of the Western Academy of Nurses that now boasted 40 members. The Academy program was "Evidence-based Practice Y2K: The Strategic Imperative" by Nancy Donaldson from the University of California San Francisco; Diane Brown from Kaiser Permanente East Bay in Walnut Creek, California; and Lowell Wise from Stanford Hospital and Clinics in Palo Alto, California (WIN, 2000). Beverly Hoeffer of Oregon Health and Science University and Marie Miller of the Colorado AHEC System joined the Program Committee (WIN, 2007b, p. 81).

Special speeches were in twos: Two Keynote Addresses were given, the first by Colleen Goode and a second by Barbara Valanis; two State of the Science symposia, one on women's health care across the lifespan and one on symptom management research; and two Distinguished Research Lectureships by Leona Eggert and Virginia Tilden. The trend in the discipline was evidence-based practice, and this concept was evident. The Keynote speeches addressed "Building on a Legacy of Excellence in Nursing Research: Evidence-Based Practice" and "Thinking Downstream: Research to Guide Evidence-Based Practice in Managed Care" respectively (WIN, 2000).

Health Care Challenges Beyond 2001: Mapping the Journey for Research and Practice – **Seattle, Washington**
In 2001, WIN partnered with the Hartford Institute for Geriatric Nursing to grant the Regional Gerontological Nursing Research Award to senior researcher Patricia Archbold at Oregon Health and Science University and new researcher Linda R. Phillips at the University of Arizona (personal communication from P. McNeil, October 4, 2016; WIN, 2007b, p. 46). This marked the beginning of a collaborative award between the Hartford Foundation and WIN to foster and showcase geriatric nursing research. Since then, 12 senior researchers and 14 new researchers have been honored (see Appendix J).

As in the previous year, major speeches were given in couples. Two Keynotes were featured: the first by Mary Blegen from the University of Colorado on nurse staffing for quality of care, and the second by Betty Gallucci from the University of Washington on genomics and pharmacogenetics. The State of the Science symposium featured two sessions: one on "Research Training: Nursing Care for Older People and Populations" by Patricia Archbold, Barbara Stewart, and Beverly Hoeffer from Oregon Health Sciences University. The second session was on "Community-based Intervention Research: Lessons Learned and Thoughts on the State of the Science" by Linda Phillips from the University of Arizona. Terry Badger of the University of Arizona became a new member of the Planning Committee, and Margaret Heitkemper was named Chair of the WIN Board of Governors (WIN, 2007b, p. 81).

2002: *Health Disparities: Meeting the Challenge* – **Palm Springs, California**
The same year that the Institute of Medicine released its report, *Unequal Treatment: Confronting Racial and Ethnic Disparities in Health Care* (IOM, 2002), WIN adopted "health disparities" as the theme of the conference. The Keynote speaker was Yvonne Maddox, Acting Deputy Director of the National Institutes of Health (NIH). State of the Science speakers extended the theme of health disparities research: Jacquelyn Flaskerud, from the University of California Los Angeles, offered an overview of concepts, research, cultural competence, and practice; Anne McNamara, from the Arizona Hospital and Healthcare Association, addressed the issue from the perspective of the looming nursing shortage; and Clarann Weinert, from Montana State University, focused on rural nursing research (WIN, 2002). The Western Academy of Nurses presented a program that addressed issues of health disparities and vulnerable populations from the perspective of emerging initiatives of nursing clinics. Presenters were Terry Badger from the University of Arizona, Aaron Strehlow from the UCLA School of Nursing Health Center at the Union Rescue Mission, Betty Gale from Arizona State University, and Sharon Howard from the Cascade County Adult Detention Center in Great Falls, Montana (personal communication, E. Nichols, February 17, 2017). Kathleen Dracup, as the Distinguished Research Lecturer, further expanded the concept of health disparities in looking "beyond the patient" to "caring for families" (WIN, 2002).

A perusal of the titles of symposia indicate that nurse researchers in the West were addressing a vast range of significant issues in health care across a growing range of populations. Following are examples: "An Emerging Contextual Model of Suffering," "Biological Markers of Injury and Related Responses," "Nurse Educator Entrepreneurs and Marginalized Populations," "One Community's Exploration in End-of-Life-Care," " Community-Based Interventions," "Nursing Systems Research," Health Disparities in Vulnerable Women and Families," and reports on cultural context of vulnerable populations, access to care in rural communities, and a report on the first five years of the California Nursing Outcomes Coalition database (see WIN, 2002).

New members of the Program Committee included Mary Blegen of the University of Colorado Health Sciences Center and Alice Tse of the University of Hawaii Manoa, with the return of Adeline Nyamathi (WIN, 2007b, p. 82).

2003: *Responding to Societal Imperatives through Discovery and Innovation* – Scottsdale, Arizona and
2004: *Hallmarks of Quality: Generating and Using Knowledge* – Portland, Oregon
The conferences of the years that immediately followed the September 11, 2001 terrorist attacks on America reinforced love and respect for each other as friends, colleagues, and members of WIN and renewed a commitment to "care deeply about those most vulnerable in our society" (McNeil, 2003). Shock and grief returned before the meetings in 2003 that followed the slayings of three members of the faculty at the University of Arizona on October 29, 2002. A nursing student took the lives of Cheryl McGaffic, Barbara Monroe, and Robin Rogers (Gabrielson, 2002; Hsiao, 2003). The theme of "Responding to Societal Imperatives" took larger meaning in the face of these tragic losses.

Geraldine (Polly) Bednash, Executive Director of the American Association of Colleges of Nursing, opened the 2003 conference on the theme of "Responding to Societal Imperatives." She was followed by State-of-Science papers by Ginette Pepper on "The Societal Imperative of Patient Safety" and Diana Wilkie on "Measurement of Pain as a Multi-Dimensional, Subjective Phenomenon."

The program committee for 2003 included Chair, Marie Driever, Terry Badger, Mary Blegen, Tina DeLapp, Beverly Hoeffer, Martha Lentz, Adeline Nyamathi, and Alice Tse (WIN, 2003). Welcomed to the Program Committee in 2004 were Marie Lobo, University of New Mexico, and Barbara Mandleco of Brigham Young University, Utah. Kay Chafey, Montana State University, was Chair of the WIN Board of Governors (WIN, 2007b, p. 83). In 2003, the focus was on "social imperatives" and in 2004 on quality in health care, both social movements in the nation. Again, in concert with recent reports from the Institute of Medicine on issues of quality in health care (see IOM, 2000; 2001; 2003; 2004a; 2004b), the committee titled the 2004 conference on a theme of quality. Quality and safety had emerged as significant issues in all aspects of the dialogue on health care.

The conference continued to grow in number of participants and complexity of structure, with several "firsts" in 2004. The first jointly funded Sigma Theta Tau International/WIN small research grant was awarded to Danuta Wojnar, a doctoral student from the University of Washington. As of 2016, 12 researchers have received a joint STTI/WIN grant. A Leadership Development Institute Initiative was launched at the 2004 conference. Also, the first poster awards, based on volunteer judges' evaluations during the conference poster sessions, were made to individual and student members (WIN, 2007b, p. 47). WIN also joined a collaboration with the Northwest Educational Outreach Network (NEON), a project funded by the U. S. Department of Education, and established the NursingPhD.org website (WIN, 2007b, p. 47).

Keynote messages were given by Marie Cowan from the University of California Los Angeles and Marita Titler from the University of Iowa Hospitals and Clinics. Their themes were generating, using, and translating knowledge. State of Science presentations were by JoAnn Congdon and Kathy Magilvy on research on long-term care and Christine Miaskowski on interventions for cancer pain as models for behavioral research. Pamela Mitchell was the Distinguished Research Lecturer on biobehavioral nursing research (WIN, 2004). All these indicated the growth of nursing research in the past decade toward quality of care and human responses in health and illness, expanding the science that defines nursing (see ANA, 2017).

A New Collaboration with WICHE: NEXus

In 2004, WIN formed a new collaboration with the Western Interstate Commission on Higher Education (WICHE) and its WCET (Western Consortium on Educational Technology), funded by a grant from the Fund for the Improvement of Postsecondary Education (FIPSE). The goal of the partnership was to increase the capacity in the West for doctoral programs in nursing by collaborative exchanges. It began with a focus on Ph.D. offerings. The project was called "The Nursing Education Xchange" (NEXus). The Founding Members were the schools of nursing of Oregon Health and Science University, the University of Colorado Denver, the University of Northern Colorado, and the University of Utah (NEXus, 2016).

The NEXus program was expanded to include courses in doctor of nursing practice (DNP) programs in 2009, with additional funding from the U. S. Health Resources and Services Administration (HRSA). It worked as an exchange of courses taught by distance modes across institutions with tuition rates "split among teaching and home institutions." By 2016, the list of academic collaborator member institutions had expanded beyond the West and included the following: Arizona State University, Case Western Reserve University, Loma Linda University, Oregon Health and Science University, The Ohio State University, University of Iowa, University of Texas Tyler, State University of New York at Buffalo, University of Colorado, University of Hawaii Manoa, University of Kansas, University of Nevada Las Vegas, University of New Mexico, University of Northern Colorado, University of Utah, Virginia Commonwealth University, and Washington State University. Academic affiliate member institutions were Idaho State University, and University of Oklahoma (NEXus, 2016).

Though the goal of NEXus was to address a nursing faculty shortage by increasing access to doctoral education, it also contributed to the advancement of research by its focus on advanced preparation that would include training in research. Its founders may not have considered it as a nod to its historical foundation, but its concept harkens to the original history of WICHE and the Western Council on Higher Education for Nursing (WCHEN) of the past: (1) It offered a cooperative exchange across states for graduate preparation of health care professionals, reflecting the original mission of WICHE (see WICHE, 2016) and (2) it served as a means for faculty development in nursing research through formal preparation, which was among the earliest priorities of WCHEN (see Chapter 2; Lindeman, 1992). NEXus has continued to be a successful model for doctoral education and continues in its twelfth year now self-supporting (Conley, et al., 2015; McNeil & Lindeman, in press).

2005: *Looking Ahead: Innovations in Nursing Science, Practice, and Education* – **San Francisco, California**
The "firsts" continued in 2005 with the jointly funded American Nurses Foundation/WIN small research grant. Also, the Biological Nursing Research Award was created and funded by Patsy A. Perry "to recognize outstanding biological research conducted by nurses." The Perry Award honors doctoral students or post-doctoral researchers focusing on physiological phenomena, with the first award going to Angela Starkweather of Washington State University in Spokane (WIN, 2007b, p. 58). As of 2016, six researchers have received this award (See Appendix K).

Melanie Dreher from Rush University opened the 2005 conference on the topic of "Redesigning Nursing Education." Three State of the Science papers addressed unique aspects of the theme of innovation: Colleen Goode, from University of Colorado Hospital, spoke on "The Science Related to the Work Environment in Acute Care Hospitals;" Marlaine Smith, University of Colorado Denver and Health Sciences Center, spoke on "Complementary-Alternative Therapies;" and Karen Thomas, from the University of Washington spoke on "Innovations in Neonatal Research."

Terry Badger, from the University of Arizona, was President of the WIN Board of Governors. Mary Blegen of the University of Colorado Health Sciences Center, Beverly Hoeffer of Oregon Health and Science University, and Alice Tse of the University of Hawaii Manoa returned to the Program Committee (2007b, p. 83).

2006: *Building Knowledge for Practice* – **Albuquerque, New Mexico**
The conference in 2006 followed the lead of its title. The special papers and award papers all related in some way to application or translation of nursing research into practice. Practice outcomes had become an increasing focus in the 2000s.

Bernadette Melnyk, from Arizona State University, gave the Keynote Address titled "Transforming Health Care from the Inside Out: Knowledge to Advance Evidence-Based Practice in Clinical and Educational Settings." State of Science papers were by Lauren Clark from the University of Colorado Denver and Health Sciences Center on early childhood obesity in Latino families and by Anne Rosenfeld from Oregon Health and Science University on improving women's cardiovascular health. Christine Miaskowski from the University of California San Francisco was awarded the Distinguished Research Lectureship and gave a history of lessons learned as a nurse scientist. The Western Academy of Nurses gave a program on the power of nursing outcome databases. Presenters were Nancy Donaldson from the University of California San Francisco, Linda Bolton from Cedar Sinai Medical Center in Los Angeles, California, and Lori Loan from Madigan Army Medical Center in Tacoma, Washington (WIN, 2006).

Judy Berg, from the University of Arizona; Barbara Mandleco, from Brigham Young University; and Adeline Nyamathi, from the University of California Los Angeles returned to the Program Committee (2007b, p. 84).

2007: *50 years of Advancing Nursing in the West* – Portland, Oregon
The "golden year" of the 50th anniversary of WCHEN/WIN was 2007. A record 200 papers were given: 108 podium presentations and 18 symposia, 128 posters, and 82 projects featured in the Research and Information Exchange (see WIN, 2007a). The focus was not on the past 50 years, but on the challenges of the future (McNeil, 2007). Nevertheless, the celebration featured the traditional *Anniversary Book* as a reminder of the unique heritage of the organization. It included reproductions of the original *Winds of Change* by Pearl Coulter; the original *Charter* of the Western Council on Higher Education for Nursing (WCHEN) of the Western Interstate Commission for Higher Education (WICHE); a chronology of major events; a list of WICHE, WCHEN, and WIN projects, conferences, and surveys; a list of award winners, members of governing boards and conference planning committees, administrative and staff support personnel. Three landmark works presented at previous conferences were reprinted: "The Research Critique: Nature, Function, and Art" by Madeleine Leininger in 1968, "Discipline of Nursing: Structure and Relationship to Practice" by Sue Donaldson and Dorothy Crowley in 1977, and "Advancing Nursing Science: Qualitative Approaches" by Jeanne Benoliel (2007b). Adding to the celebration, the dissertation award was established in conjunction with the Council on the Advancement of Nursing Science (CANS) (WIN, 2007b, p. 47).

The meetings began with unique keynote panels and respondents. The Education Keynote and Panel included Christine Tanner, from Oregon Health and Science University with response by Carol Ashton from Idaho State University and commentary by Patricia Benner from the University of California San Francisco. The Practice Keynote Panel included Marie Driever from Providence Portland Medical Center; Julie McNulty from Alaska Native Medical Center and doctoral student at Oregon Health and Science University; Nancy Nowak from Intermountain Healthcare in Salt Lake City, Utah, and Lorie Wild from the University of Washington Medical Center. The Research Keynote and Panel featured Margaret Heitkemper from the University of Washington, with respondents Cindy Mendelson from the University of New Mexico and Adeline Nyamathi from the University of California Los Angeles. Maureen Keefe was honored with the Distinguished Research Lecture on "Coming of Age in the Western Institute of Nursing" (WIN, 2007a).

The Western Academy of Nurses Panel featured "50th Anniversary Challenge Papers" on Education, by Roberta Everson from Washington State University and Kathie Records from Arizona State University. The paper on Practice was given by Joachim Voss from the University of Washington, and the challenge paper on research was given by Martha Driessnack from the University of Iowa (WIN, 2007a).

Members of the Golden Anniversary committee were Chair Donna Velasquez of Arizona; Marie Cowan, California; Tina DeLapp, Alaska; Jo Eleanor Elliott, Colorado; Barbara Gaines, Oregon; Carol Lindeman, California; Jeanne Kearns, Colorado; Ginette Pepper, Utah; Jackie Pflaum, Alaska; Bryce Strang, Oregon; and Paula McNeil of WIN. The members of the Board of Governors at the time were President Ginette Pepper, Utah; President-Elect Marty Lentz, Washington; Secretary-Treasurer Paula Meek, New Mexico; Governor-at-large Tina DeLapp, Alaska; Governor Representative of Nursing Education Judy Berg, Arizona; Governor Representative of Nursing Practice Marie J. Driever, Oregon; Governor Representative of Nursing Research Marie Lobo, New Mexico; and Student ex officio, Allison Webel, California (WIN, 2007b, p. vi). The Program Committee, chaired by Marie Driever, welcomed new members Lauren Clark, University of Colorado at Denver and Health Science

Center; Lori Loan, Madigan Army Medical Center, Washington; Patricia Pearce, University of Utah; and Karen Zulkowski, Montana State University. Ginnette Pepper, from the University of Utah, was President (note change of designation from "Chair") of the WIN Board of Governors (WIN, 2007b, p. 84).

2008: *The Circle of Nursing Knowledge: Education, Practice, and Research* – **Garden Grove, California and**
2009: *Networks in Nursing Science: Creating Our Future* - **Salt Lake City, Utah**
A general underlying theme of the conferences of the next five years was the integration and collaboration of nurses and other health care professionals and their work in education, practice, and research. This was reflected in the Keynote speech by Pamela Mitchell in 2008. She framed the topic of integration of research, practice, and education from the perspectives of translational research into practice, practice into research from a practice-based evidence model, and incorporation of research concepts into nursing curricula (Mitchell, 2008, pp. 3-7).

Other special papers in 2008 included State of the Science presentations by Cecily Betz from the University of Southern California on "Health Care Transitions of Youth with Special Health Care Needs," Jean Giddens from the University of New Mexico on "Virtual Experiential Communities" in nursing education, and Linda Phillips from the University of California Los Angeles on "Culturally Competent Care for Persons with Chronic Illness." Clarann Weinert was awarded the Distinguished Research Lectureship. Marilyn Chow, from Kaiser Permanente in Oakland, California, represented the Western Academy of Nurses on "Translating Research Findings into Everyday Clinical Practice" (WIN, 2008).

In 2009, the first Ann M. Voda American Indian/Alaskan Native/First Nation Conference Award was given to Molly Butler Aultz of Oregon Health and Science University. The award is sponsored by Ann Voda to allow an American Indian, Alaska Native or First Nation student or clinician to attend the conference. As of 2016, seven students have received the award to begin engagement in WIN (See Appendix L).

Another "first" in 2009 was the Keynote presentation that listed two authors from the University of Washington. Margaret Heitkemper, from the School of Nursing, introduced Mary (Nora) Disis, from the School of Medicine. She gave an informative description, explanation, and model case of The Clinical and Translational Science Awards (CTSAs) at the National Center of Research at NIH. This initiative began with a consortium of 38 academic health centers in 23 states (8 of which are located in 5 western states). The purposes are the following:

1. Improve the way biomedical research is conducted across the country.
2. Reduce the time it takes for laboratory discoveries to become treatments for patients.
3. Engage communities in clinical research efforts.
4. Train the next generation of clinical and translational researchers.

This mechanism opened a new approach with the goal to "get new treatments more efficiently and quickly to patients" (Heitkemper & Disis, 2009, p. 3). It also continued a new era for nursing research collaboration in a multidisciplinary environment. Finally, it began the conference on the theme of "networks" from a unique and important perspective.

The other special papers of 2009 reflected new directions in methods at the leading edge of multi-disciplinary science. State of Science papers introduced practice-based evidence in contrast to evidence-based practice by Susan Horn from the Institute for Clinical Outcomes Research in Salt Lake City, Utah; Deborah Koniak-Griffin, from the University of California Los Angeles, introduced methods to "[Partner] with Consumers to Design Health Promotion Research;" and Christine Miaskowski from the University of California San Francisco and Paula Meek from the University of Colorado Denver described "Opportunities and Challenges in Symptom Clusters Research" (WIN, 2009).

The Western Academy of Nurses Program completed the unique focus on "networks" with a program on partnerships in education and practice. Terry Badger from the University of Arizona, Susan Beck from the University of Utah, Patricia Horoho from Madigan Army Medical Center in Tacoma Washington, and Joanne Warner from the University of Portland outlined several initiatives in such partnerships. They included the accelerated degree program, the dedicated education unit in the clinical setting, the Veteran's Affairs Nursing Academies, and the Army Nurse Corps Human Capital Campaign (WIN, 2009, p. 61).

Presidents of the WIN Board of Governors during 2008 and 2009 were Ginette Pepper, from the University of Utah, and Martha Lentz, from the University of Washington, respectively. Program Committee members were Marie Driever, Chair, from Group Health Cooperative in Seattle, Washington; Marie Lobo, from the University of New Mexico; Judy Berg, from the University of Arizona; Lauren Clark, from the University of Utah; Tina DeLapp, from the University of Alaska; Margaret Heitkemper and Martha Lentz, from the University of Washington, and Lori Loan, from Madigan Army Medical Center in Tacoma, Washington; Barbara Mandleco, Brigham Young University, Utah; and Patricia Pearce, University of Utah (WIN, 2008, p. 537; WIN 2009, p. xxvi).

In December, 2008, WIN tragically lost two of its members. Carol Macnee and Susan McCabe, faculty and researchers at the University of Wyoming, were killed in an automobile accident as they were traveling together in northern Colorado (The Denver Channel, 2008). They were co-authors of the book, *Understanding Nursing Research*. Macnee was Director of Research at the School of Nursing in Wyoming, and McCabe was in the midst of projects on health of rural women and learning experiences of Psychiatric Mental Health Nurse Practitioner students (Pine & Burman, 2009). They had each presented at the *Communicating Nursing Research* conference three times.

The Affordable Care Act Changes Access to Health Care and Research Issues in the United States

On March 23, 2010, the Patient Protection and Affordable Care Act (PPACA), Affordable Care Act (ACA), called "Obamacare," was signed into law. This changed insurance coverage and subsequent access to health care for many United States citizens. Several aspects of the Act were implemented across time, with some terms in law as late as January 1, 2014. Generally, with few exceptions, the Act mandated health insurance coverage for all citizens. It provided for state exchanges or expansion of Medicaid to allow people without health insurance to obtain coverage. Further, it provided that health insurance companies could not refuse coverage for pre-existing conditions, allowed parents to keep children on their health insurance until the age of 26 years, gave the right to appeal when an insurance company declines coverage, disallowed insurance companies from cancelling coverage for honest mistakes in applications, called for no annual or lifetime limits of coverage, and provided for preventive care at no additional cost. In addition, the Act required health care providers to document effectiveness in positive health outcomes and safety in order to be reimbursed for care (Health Network Group, 2017; HHS, 2017).

The advent of the ACA stimulated discussion among health care professionals regarding implications of care, especially related to nursing interventions. Calls for outcome measurement and documentation, assurance of patient safety, and potential increasing needs for primary care and preventive services both inspired and mandated new ideas for translation and practice research. The ACA and other national initiatives and reports, including several reports from the Institute of Medicine influenced the entire profession of nursing and the themes and direction of discussion at the *Communicating Nursing Research* conference in the West.

Indeed, Heather Young later observed:

While the ACA does little to address education and research directly, there is no question that sweeping change in health care delivery will precipitate new demands on education, both for retooling health professionals and for addressing projected workforce shortages related to growing demand and shrinking supply . . . We will need more, and better educated, nurses to practice in new ways and in different and more complex settings, with more diverse populations (Young, 2013, p. 4).

2010: *Nursing Science: Informing Practice and Driving Policy* – Glendale, Arizona and
2011: *Transitions: Unifying Practice, Education, and Research to Improve Health* – Las Vegas, Nevada
The years of 2010 and 2011 were especially important to WIN and to the discipline. The theme of the 2010 conference was nursing engagement in policy, reflecting a growing national interest in the profession as it responded to national and societal imperatives. At the end of 2010, the Institute of Medicine (IOM) released its first report on the profession, *The Future of Nursing: Leading Change, Advancing Health* (IOM, 2011). WIN members, Linda Bolton and Michael Bleich were on the Committee of the Robert Wood Johnson Foundation Initiative on the Future of Nursing at the IOM that contributed to the report; and Heather Young was listed as an official reviewer of the report. Key recommendations were the following:

1. Nurses should practice to the full extent of their education and training.
2. Nurses should achieve higher levels of education and training through an improved education system that promotes seamless academic progression.
3. Nurses should be full partners, with physicians and other health professionals, in redesigning health care in the United States.
4. Effective workforce planning and policy making require better data collection and an improved information infrastructure (IOM, 2011).

Each of these areas invited new thinking, innovation, and collaboration in nursing education, practice, and research. They became topics of presentations and discussions at the conferences.

Given the national attention to nursing, the 2010 Keynote Address at the *Communicating Nursing Research* conference was fitting to be offered by Nancy Ridenour, Dean of the University of New Mexico and Robert Wood Johnson Fellow in Health Policy Alumna. Her address was "Integrating Practice, Research, and Education with Policy" (personal communication from M. Lobo, February 15, 2017). State of the Science papers were offered by Paul Cook, from the University of Colorado Denver, on "Research, Program Evaluation, or QI? Mapping the Edges in Adherence Studies;" Janice Morse, from the University of Utah, on "Towards Establishing a Qualitative Evidence;" and Huong Nguyen, from the University of Washington, on "Digital Health Consumers: Transforming the Clinical Research Landscape" (WIN, 2010). Ginette Pepper, from the University of Utah, delivered the Distinguished Research Lectureship, exploring a career of building bridges across the gaps between "diverse disciplinary perspectives, mind-body dichotomy, service and education, and the quality chasm" (Pepper, 2010, p. 47-58). The Western Academy of Nurses program focused on outcomes of hospital magnet designation (WIN, 2010).

Even beyond recent IOM reports, the health care environment at this time was ripe for education, practice, and/or research organizations to re-examine their missions. Advances in technology had allowed data collection and analysis of patient care experiences, interventions, outcomes, and costs. Initiatives adopted in the past decade within health care systems and among research communities had blurred some lines between research and quality improvement. Examples of such enterprises included the Triple Aim ("improve patient care experience, improve the health of a population, reduce per capita health care costs") (IHI, 2017) and improvement science (ISRN, 2017). These concepts had emerged among WIN Assembly and *Communicating Nursing Research* presentations.

In 2011, the WIN Board of Governors adopted new Mission, Vision, and Goals. Compared with the previous functions of the Charter of the Western Council on Higher Education for Nursing (WCHEN) (see Chapter 1) and the WIN mission and goals at its advent in 1986 (see Chapter 4), the research mission now returned to a central and integrated part of WIN, rather than part of the separate mission of the Western Society for Research in Nursing (WSRN). It is also interesting to note the use of contemporary trends, style, and jargon in each mission (i.e. in 1957: "functions" rather than goals, and deference to "the Commission;" in 1986: "promote proactive stances," and "strong regional voice;" and in 2011: "health outcomes" [rather than simply "health"], use of the words "science" and "scholarship"). The mission statements are compared in Table 5-1.

Also in 2011, WIN partnered again with the John A. Hartford Foundation to offer the Regional Geriatric Nursing Education Award, following the partnered Regional Geriatric Nursing Research Award established in 2001. The first recipient of the Education award was Catherine Van Son from Washington State University in Spokane (See Appendix M).

The Keynote Address in 2011 was given by Michael Bleich, from Oregon Health and Science University, and focused on the recent IOM report on *The Future of Nursing*

Table 5-1. Comparison of WCHEN/WIN Function/Mission Statements:1957, 1986, and 2011

1957	1986	2011
Charter	**Mission**	**Mission**
The Western Interstate Commission for Higher Education (hereinafter referred to as the Commission), recognizing the need for regional development of graduate education and research in nursing, has authorized the organization of a planning group to be known as the Western Council on Higher Education for Nursing [WCHEN].	The mission of WIN is to influence positively the quality of health care for people in the West through monitoring relevant issues and trends and through designing, implementing, and evaluating regional action-oriented nursing strategies in nursing education, nursing practice, and nursing research.	The Western Institute of Nursing exists to bring together a diverse community of nurses in a shared commitment to advance nursing science, education, and practice to improve health outcomes. **Vision** The Western Institute of Nursing: Leading Nursing Research, Education, and Practice
Functions Recommend to the Commission policies relating to graduate education and research in nursing. Provide a medium for exchange of ideas and sharing of experiences by Western institutions of higher learning which offer programs of education for professional nursing. Undertake cooperative planning for nursing education programs within the Western region under the auspices of the Commission. Identify problems with respect to nursing education which need cooperative study Stimulate research in nursing within colleges and universities of the Western region (see Coulter, 1963, p. 25; WCHEN, 1957, p. 63; WIN, 1992, p. 10, WIN, 2007b, pp. 27-36).	**Goals** Promote proactive stances to health care issues and trends which foster the partnership between nursing practice and nursing education; Promote a strong regional voice and network for nursing in the West; Promote quality nursing educational programs that are responsive to the evolving needs of the health are livery system; Promote quality nursing practice through innovative approaches to the delivery of health care; Facilitate the development of nurse leaders; Monitor and project requirements for nursing in the West, based on societal trends and health care issues; Promote strong regional societies which promote improvement or advancement of nurses and nursing (WIN 2007b, pp. 44-45).	**Goals*** Provide forums for the exchange of scholarship and research. Stabilize and expand funding sources in order to meet financial goals. Encourage the application of evidence-based practice. Encourage the incorporation of meritorious research in nursing curricula. Facilitate WIN having a voice in health care policy deliberations and formulation. *Specific strategic activities (1 to 6 in number) were listed under each goal (See WIN, 2011b).

(see IOM, 2011). State of Science papers also addressed current issues in the discipline. They were given by Amy Barton, from the University of Colorado; Nancy Staggers, from the University of Maryland; and Joyce Verran, from the University of Colorado. Topics were quality and safety, effectiveness in the case of nursing handoffs in acute care settings, and research methods for complexity. The Distinguished Research Lecturer was Bernadette Melnyk from Arizona State University, who described the latest science related to evidence-based practice (WIN, 2011).

Martha Lentz continued as President of the WIN Board of Governors, replaced by Marie Driever from Oregon and Washington in 2011. Program Committee members were Judith Berg from Arizona and California, Lauren Clark from Utah, Tina DeLapp from Alaska, Margaret Heitkemper and Martha Lentz from Washington, Anne Marie Kotzer from Colorado, Lori Loan from Washington, Marie Lobo from New Mexico, Barbara Mandleco from Utah, Jan Schultz from Hawaii, Donna Velasquez from Arizona, and Karen Zulkowski, from Montana (WIN, 2010; 2011).

The conference expanded beyond the scope of management for its volunteer organizers among members of WIN and support staff. By 2010, the conference had expanded its staff to include a professional conference planner, Bo Perry (personal communication from M. Lobo, February 15, 2017).

A New Standard for Growth in *Communicating Nursing Research*
The years of 2012 through 2016 showed unprecedented growth in the number of presenters at the Conference. Total number of papers presented averaged 221 for those years. The average for the previous five years was 190, a 16 percent increase. Average numbers of presenters during the five years of 2012 through 2016 compared with the previous five years are shown in Table 5-2.

Table 5-2. Comparison of 5-Year Averages of Participants in *Communicating Nursing Research*		
2007-2011	2012-2016	Percent Increase
Average of Total Number of Papers Presented from Submitted Abstracts		
190	221	16%
Average Number of Podium Presentations		
100	120	20%
Average Number of Symposia		
18	20	10%
Average Number of Posters		
182	405	223%
Average Number of Projects in Research Information Exchange		
106	162	53%

These figures would have likely been beyond even the most optimistic dreams of the pioneers who began the conference in 1968 with five papers.

Advancing to National and Global Perspectives

McNeil and Lindeman (in press) note that technology advancements allowed the expansion of the conference and its influence to national and global audiences, which is true, but the continuing innovation, improvement, and high expectations of quality saw their fruits in the increasing stature of the conference.

2012: *Advancing Scientific Innovations in Nursing* – Portland, Oregon

In 2012, the special sessions offered a model case of innovation in thinking, questions, methods, and use of outcomes. They were exemplars in the positive growth of the discipline and its science. Kathi Mooney, from the University of Utah, gave the Keynote Address on the conference theme of scientific innovations. Three State of the Science papers included Gary Donaldson from the Pain Research Center of the University of Utah, who challenged current practices in randomized trials for comparative effectiveness; Diane Skiba from the University of Colorado, who examined the influence of social media in health care; and Kathleen Stevens from the University of Texas Health Science Center San Antonio, who described the state of the work in the area of improvement science. Martha Lentz gave the Distinguished Lecture, tracking her career work on sleep research. The Carol Lindeman New Researcher, Terri Yost, and the Pat Perry Biological Nursing Research Awardee, Charles Downs, offered uniquely innovative views of intervention for mild traumatic brain injury and changes in telomeres of lung alveolar cells related to cigarette smoke. The Western Academy of Nurses Panel featured a discussion by Deborah Koniak-Griffin and Kynna Wright-Volel from the University of California Los Angeles, Janna Lesser from the University of Texas Health Science Center San Antonio, and Usha Menon from Arizona State University on community-based participatory research as a strategy to decrease health inequities (WIN, 2012).

Marie Driever was President of the WIN Board of Governors. New members added to the Program Committee were Doris Boutain from the University of Washington, Jennifer Mensik from St. Luke's Regional Medical Center, Boise, Idaho, and Charlene Winters from Montana State University (WIN, 2012, p. xxxii).

2013: *Creating a Shared Future of Nursing: Research, Practice, and Education* – Anaheim, California and
2014: *Taking it Global: Research, Practice, and Education in Nursing* – Seattle, Washington

The themes of the meetings of 2013 and 2014 further indicated that nursing and nursing research in the West were moving into the future, collaborating across the country, and across the world. A significant number of papers were presented by researchers from across the United States and many countries of the world.

The 2013 Keynote speaker Heather Young, from the University of California Davis, described the "Campaign for Action," an initiative to activate coalitions of "policymakers, health care professionals, educators, and business leaders" in every state to "respond to the country's increasing demand for safe, high-quality, and effective health care" and to "improve America's health through nursing." The daunting initiative is sponsored by the Robert Wood Johnson Foundation, the American Association of Retired Persons (AARP), and the AARP Foundation. This work is in response to the IOM report on *The Future of Nursing* (Campaign for Action, 2017; IOM, 2011). Young shared the specific actions of coalitions in each of the 13 member states of WIN (WIN, 2013).

Young's speech was stirring and reminiscent of the tone and zeal of the early WIN pioneers, as she channeled Coulter's *The Winds of Change* (Coulter, 1963) and Elliott's parting words to the National League for Nursing:

If you are feeling that the sands beneath your feet are shifting, *the winds of change are at gale force*, and your comfortable assumptions about your roles and resources are threatened, you are not alone! I cannot imagine a better time for nurses to lead change and advance health. The good news is that *for the first time, a concerted national effort* is underway to take advantage of the uncertainty and to forge ahead with new solutions that will transform healthcare and secure rational paths towards improved population health [emphasis added] (Young, 2013, p. 3).

One could almost see pioneers like Pearl Coulter proclaiming "the winds of change," the Committees of Seven creating "for the first time, a concerted [regional] effort" and Jo Eleanor Elliott challenging in her inspiring style, "Helmets down, lances up, full speed ahead" (Bak, 2011).

Young's speech was followed by State of the Science Papers by Maureen Keefe from the University of Utah, on trends and innovations in nursing education; Joan Shaver, on biobehavioral nursing science; and Marla Weston and Cheryl Peterson from the American Nurses Association, and Kathleen White from Johns Hopkins School of Nursing. They spoke on implications for nursing into the future following *The Future of Nursing*, IOM report (2011) and the passage of the ACA (WIN, 2013).

The following year, 2014, the conference truly "took it Global," creating an unprecedented view of health and human needs as well as nursing initiatives in developing and low-resource countries. David Shoultz, from the Bill and Melinda Gates Foundation, opened the meeting on "Nursing and Health: A Global Perspective," expanding the vision of WIN members far beyond the region or the nation.

R. Kevin Mallinson, from George Mason University in Fairfax, Virginia, continued on the topic of strengthening nursing practice in "low-resource countries." He shared insights from his experiences in Lesotho, South Africa and the Kingdom of Swaziland, with a focus on the work in Sub Saharan Africa. He observed:

For many of us in the United States, it is an exciting time to be a nurse! We have access to the best of technology, all the information one could want through the worldwide web, clean and relatively safe workplaces, and innumerable, cheap options for continuing education programs. We have ample opportunities to improve our practice and maximize the outcomes for our patients or enrich the education of our students. And our reputation as 'nurses' remains excellent . . . (Mallinson, 2014).

Adeline Nyamathi, from the University of California Los Angeles, followed with a report on a decade of nursing research on global issues of malaria; tuberculosis; HIV/AIDS; women, children, and reproductive health; and gender-based violence in post conflict settings. She concluded by outlining challenges in designing research in countries abroad and "developing a road map for the next decade" (Nyamathi, 2014, p. 21).

Joachim Voss, from the University of Washington, extended the world health focus with impressive examples of innovation in nursing education at Makarere University in Uganda and Khon Kaen University in Thailand. He also described the Afya Bora Global Health Leadership Training consortium. The group includes faculty from medicine, nursing, and public health from four universities in the United States (University of Washington, University of California San Francisco, Johns Hopkins University, and University of Pennsylvania) and African partners of University of Nairobi Kenya, Muhimbili University Tanzania, Makarere University Uganda, and University of Botswana (Voss, 2014).

The Panel of the Western Academy of Nurses followed the theme with "Research Innovations in Global Health Nursing." Participants were Joanne Whitney, Sarah Gimbel, and Pamela Kohler from the University of Washington, joined by Mary Anne Mercer, Technical Advisor for the Timor-Leste program of the Health Alliance International in Seattle, and Julia Robinson, Deputy Director of Cote d'Ivoire programs of Health Alliance International in Seattle, Washington.

Judith Berg was President of the WIN Board of Governors. Program Committee members were Lauren Clark from the University of Utah; Barbara Mandleco from Brigham Young University; Doris Boutain, Martha Lentz, and Lori Loan from the University of Washington; Tina DeLapp from the University of Alaska, Marie Driever from Oregon and Washington, clinical research consultant, Teresa Goodell from Oregon Health and Science University, Margo Halm from Salem (Oregon) Health, Anne Marie Kotzer from the University of Colorado, Marie Lobo from the University of New Mexico, Jennifer Mensik from St. Luke's Boise and Meridian Medical Centers (Idaho), Roberta Rehm and Kathryn Lee from California, Jan Shoultz from Hawaii, Donna Velasquez from Arizona, and Charlene Winters from Montana (WIN, 2013; 2014).

2015: *Equity and Access: Nursing Research, Practice, and Education* – Albuquerque, New Mexico
2016: *Innovations in Engagement through Research Practice, and Education* – Anaheim, California
If any unifying themes were to describe the conferences of the years of 2015 and 2016, they would likely be extraordinary growth in participation, increasing diversity of participants, and a commitment to the tripartite mission of nursing research, practice, and education to improve health care. Indeed half of the titles of the conference of the past decade included the three words "research, practice, and education," reflecting the same consistency on the WCHEN/WIN logo. Presentations spanned issues in the discipline of nursing in the broadest sense.

Keynote speakers both in 2015 and 2016 were not nurses. In 2015, Barbara Safriet, from the Lewis and Clark Law School in Portland, Oregon, spoke to the conference theme on "Equity and Access: Melding Policy with Nursing Research, Practice, and Education." The following year, George Demiris, from the University of Washington, spoke on "Informatics Tools for Patient Engagement." Conferences of both years featured a range of diversity in State of Science papers. Presenters were Paula Gubrud from Oregon Health and Science University; Sandra Haldane from the Alaska Native Tribal Health Consortium in Anchorage, Alaska; David Vlahov from the University of California San Francisco; Debra Barksdale from Virginia Commonwealth University; Bonnie Gance-Cleveland from the University of Colorado; and Kate Lorig from the School of Medicine at Stanford University in Palo Alto, California (WIN, 2015; 2016).

Panels of the Western Academy of Nursing featured topics of key interest to nursing scholars. The first was "Emerging Opportunities for Big Data in Nursing" by John Welton and Blaine Reeder from the University of Colorado (WIN, 2015). The second topic was "Changing Landscape in the World of Publishing: What Authors Need to Know." This session featured Deborah Koniak-Griffin from the University of California Los Angeles and highly published author; Steve Clancy, Research Librarian and Bibliographer at the Ayala Science Library and Grunigen Medical Library at the University of California Irvine; Nancy Lowe, Editor-in-Chief of the *Journal of Obstetric, Gynecologic, and Neonatal Nursing (JOGNN)*; and Jan Morse, Editor of *Qualitative Health Research* and *Global Qualitative Nursing Research* (WIN, 2016).

Marie Lobo was President of the WIN Board of Governors. Program Committee members were Chair Donna Velasquez, Arizona; Judith Berg, Arizona and California; Lauren Clark and Katreena Merrill, Utah; Tina DeLapp, Alaska; Mary Ellen Dellefield, Kathryn Lee, Roberta Rehm, Anthony McGuire, Bronwyn Fields, and Annette Nasr, California; Marie Driever, Oregon and Washington; Margo Halm and Kristin Lutz, Oregon; Lori Hendrickx, South Dakota; Martha Lentz and Catherine Von Son, Washington; Lori Loan, Maryland; Marie Lobo, New Mexico; Charlene Winters, Montana; and Bonnie Gance-Cleveland, Colorado (WIN, 2015; 2016).

In 2015, the Board of Governors established a Development Committee with the following goals: (1) to raise at least $50,000 by 2017 in honor of the 50th *Communicating Nursing Research* conference, and (2) to increase the number and funding amount of research awards. Immediately, the STTI/WIN award was increased from $5,000 to $10,000, and a plan for the CANS/WIN Award for $5,000 was initiated. The ultimate goal of development was to endow a fund that would support all of the WIN awards (personal communication. M. Lobo, February 22, 2017).

Another National Report for Nursing—*Advancing Healthcare Transformation: A New Era for Academic Nursing*

In March of 2016, the American Association of Colleges of Nursing (AACN) released a landmark report, *Advancing Healthcare Transformation: A New Era for Academic Nursing.* Its purpose was to "[examine] the potential for enhanced partnership between academic nursing and academic health centers around the imperative to advance integrated systems of healthcare, achieve improved health outcomes, and foster new models for innovation" (AACN, 2016, p. 2). This appeared to complement the other major recent national reports, particularly from the Institute of Medicine, on nursing. The report began with descriptions of its major findings:

1. Academic nursing is not positioned as a partner in healthcare transformation.
2 Institutional leaders recognize the missed opportunity for alignment with academic nursing and are seeking a new approach.
3. Insufficient resources are a barrier to supporting a significantly enhanced role for academic nursing. This finding asserted that schools of nursing receive 0.4 percent of NIH funding (AACN, 2016, p. 3).

The report offered six recommendations. The similarity of these recommendations to those issues valiantly addressed by Jo Eleanor Elliott are striking. While it is true that the focus of WCHEN was on more local regional needs in nursing education and research to improve patient care, the scope of current attention for nursing has moved to a larger world view. But the fundamental areas of focus on resources, collaboration, faculty development, and research to improve education, practice, and policy continued fundamentally the same. Indeed, a review of the first regional conference programs and minutes of WCHEN meetings reveals a haunting consistency. This is an important topic for historical scholars today.

1. Embrace a new vision for academic nursing. This included the advancement of nurse participation in health system governance and collaborative workforce plans and training programs with health systems.
2. Enhance the clinical practice of academic nursing.
3. Partner in preparing the nurses of the future.
4. Partner in the implementation of accountable care.
5. Invest in nursing research programs and better integrate research into clinical practice. This recommendation included creating mechanisms to coordinate research projects and activities across academic nursing, strengthening training programs for nurses in clinical research, and providing leadership in establishing linkages to other professional schools, and expanding nursing faculty development and recruitment to include Ph.D. investigators across multiple disciplines in targeted research areas.
6. Implement an advocacy agenda in support of a new era for academic nursing.

2017: *Leadership: Continuing the Vision* - Denver, Colorado
In 2017, the *Communicating Nursing Research* conference celebrates its 50th anniversary, as well as the 60th anniversary of the Western Institute of Nursing (WIN). This writing precedes the date of the celebration, so is offered in anticipation of the event.

The conference returns to Colorado, the state of the original headquarters of the Western Interstate Council on Higher Education (WICHE), the Western Council on Higher Education for Nursing (WCHEN), and WIN. The highlight of the conference will be the return of presidential historian, Doris Kearns Goodwin. She keynoted the WIN Assembly in Albuquerque in 1991 (WIN, 1991). She was born in Oceanside, on Long Island and raised in Rockville Centre, on Long Island, New York, the sister of WIN's own Jeanne Kearns. She graduated from Colby College and earned the Ph.D. in government from Harvard University. She has written many highly acclaimed works, including presidential biographies on Lyndon Johnson, the Kennedy family, Franklin and Eleanor Roosevelt (for which she won the 1995 Pulitzer Prize for History), Theodore Roosevelt and William Howard Taft, and the honored book on Lincoln, *Team of Rivals.* Her next book will be on leadership. She is well known for her television appearances where she offers historical insights into current political events. She speaks to audiences throughout the country on aspects of history and leadership ("Doris Kearns Goodwin," 2012; 2016).

The conference will continue to feature State of the Science speakers. This year, three respected leaders will present. Linda Sarna, Dean and Professor of the University of California Los Angeles will speak on Research; Heather Young, Associate Vice Chancellor for Nursing and Dean and Professor at the University of California Davis, will speak on Education; and Susan Bakewell-Sachs, Dean and Vice President for

Nursing Affairs at Oregon Health and Science University, will speak on Practice. These three scholars have also prepared an analysis of the implications of three major initiatives discussed here: The Affordable Care Act, the Institute of Medicine Report of the *Future of Nursing,* and the report by AACN on *Advancing Healthcare Transformation.* Their work is currently in press as a follow-up article in *Nursing Research* (Young, Bakewell-Sachs, & Sarna, in press). Executive Director, Paula McNeil and long-time supporter of WIN, Carol Lindeman, also have an article on the history of WIN forthcoming in *Nursing Research* (McNeil & Lindeman, in press).

National and International Influence

Since the first conference in 1968 that focused on the needs for nursing and its public of the West, the reputation of the *Communicating Nursing Research* conference, as well as advances in technology, expanded the influence of the Western conference far beyond its borders. Indeed, there is no better example of national and international engagement of WIN than the conference program for 2017. Doris Kearns Goodwin will raise the vision even beyond nursing and provide a view of the broadest perspective of what it means to be a leader at the highest levels. Also, analysis of participants from 2013 to 2016 reveals their origins in 43 states, Washington DC, and Australia, Canada, India, Israel, Japan, Lebanon, South Korea, Spain, Taiwan, Turkey, and Uganda. The conference has continued to grow in sheer numbers. In 1968, five papers were presented. In 2016, 194 papers were presented as well as 465 posters, with a total of 926 in attendance (McNeil & Lindeman, in press).

Beyond growth in numbers, the conference continues to attract an increasingly broad interest in all aspects of nursing practice, education, and research. WIN continues to be actively engaged in the significant national and international health care issues. This includes active discussion and debate of such issues at the Conference. The future appears broad and bright for *Communicating Nursing Research.*

At this writing, with a new United States Congress and Administration who have promised to repeal and replace the current national health care legislation of the Affordable Care Act (ACA), but who have not put forth the specifics of change, only one thing can be said for certain. The present and future challenges for nursing to better serve the health care needs of all will continue to grow, and the opportunities for WIN and nursing in the West to contribute to solving these challenges will intensify.

References

American Association of Colleges of Nursing (AACN) (2016). *Advancing healthcare transformation: A new era for academic nursing.* Washington DC: AACN.

American Nurses Association (ANA). (2017). What is nursing? Retrieved February 12, 2017 from http://www.nursingworld.org/EspeciallyForYou/What-is-Nursing.

Bak, G. P. (2011, June). Jo Eleanor Elliott: A legacy of courage. *American Nurse Today, 6(6).*

Campaign for action (2017). Retrieved February 14, 2017 from http://campaignforaction.org/about/our-story/.

Conley, V. P., Heitkemper, M., McCarthy, D., Anderson, C. M., Corwin, E. J., Daack-Hirsch, S., Dorsey, S. G., Gregory, K. E., Groer, M. W., Henly, S. J., Landers, T., Lyon, D. E., Taylor, J. Y., & Voss, J. (2015). Educating future nursing scientists: Recommendations for integrating omics content in PhD programs. *Nursing Outlook, 63,* 417-427.

Coulter, P. P. (1963, July). Appendix C. In *The winds of change: Progress report of regional cooperation in collegiate nursing education in the West.* Boulder, CO: WICHE. WIN archives, Portland, OR.

Council for the Advancement of Nursing Science (CANS). (2016). Council history. Retrieved February 3, 2017 from http://www.nursingscience.org/about/council-history.

Doris Kearns Goodwin. (2012). Retrieved January 29, 2017 from http://www.doriskearnsgoodwin.com/about.html.

Doris Kearns Goodwin. (2016, May 2). Retrieved January 29, 2017 from http://www.biography.com/people/doris-kearns-goodwin-38566#other-projects-and-personal-life

Gabrielson, R. (2002, October 29). Student kills 3 professors, self. *Arizona Daily Wildcat,* 1.

Gortner, S. R. (1992). The federal role. In *The anniversary book: A history of nursing in the West 1956-1992* (pp. 63-67). Boulder, CO: WIN.

Health and Human Services. (2017). *Compilation of Patient Protection and Affordable Care Act.* Retrieved February 13, 2017 from https://www.hhs.gov/sites/default/files/ppacacon.pdf.

Health Network Group. (2017). *Obamacare facts.* Retrieved February 13, 2017 from https://obamacare.net/obamacare-facts/.

Heitkemper, M., & Disis, M. L. (2009). CTSAs: An interdisciplinary approach to improving patient care T1 translation in an academic environment: Breast cancer vaccine development. In *Communicating Nursing Research, 42; WIN Assembly 17* (pp. 1-6). Portland, OR: WIN.

Hsiao, I. (2003, May 15). Tragedy binds UA nurses-to-be. *Tucson Citizen,* 1.

Improvement Science Research Network (ISRN). (2017). *What is improvement science?* Retrieved February 14, 2017 from https://isrn.net/about/improvement_science.asp.

Institute for Healthcare Improvement (IHI). (2017). *A primer on the Triple Aim.* Retrieved February 14, 2017 from http://www.ihi.org/resources/Pages/Publications/PrimerDefiningTripleAim.aspx.

Institute of Medicine (IOM). (2000). *To err is human: Building a safer health system.* L. T. Kohn, J. M. Corrigan, & M. S. Donaldson (Eds.). Washington DC: National Academies Press.

Institute of Medicine (IOM). (2001). *Crossing the quality chasm: A new health system for the 21st century.* Washington DC: National Academies Press.

Institute of Medicine (IOM). (2002). *Unequal treatment: Confronting racial and ethnic disparities in health care.* B. D. Smedley, A. Y. Stith, & A. R. Nelson (Eds.) Washington DC: National Academies Press.

Institute of Medicine (IOM). (2003). *Health professions education: A bridge to quality.* A. C. Greiner & E. Knebel (Eds.). Washington DC: National Academies Press.

Institute of Medicine (IOM). (2004a). *Keeping patients safe: Transforming the work environment of nurses.* A. Page (Ed.). Washington DC: National Academies Press.

Institute of Medicine (IOM). (2004b). *Patient safety: Achieving a new standard for care.* P. Aspden, J. M. Corrigan, J. Wolcott, & S. M. Erickson (Eds.). Washington DC: National Academies Press.

Institute of Medicine (IOM). (2006). *Preventing medication errors.* P. Aspden, J. Wolcott, J. L. Bootman, & L. R. Cronenwett (Eds.). Washington DC: National Academies Press.

Institute of Medicine (IOM). (2011). *The future of nursing: Leading change, advancing health.* Washington DC: National Academies Press.

Kohn, L. T., Corrigan, J. M., & Donaldson, M. S. (Eds.). *To err is human: Building a safer health system.* Washington DC: Institute of Medicine of the National Academies Press.

Leininger, M. (1992). Reflections on WCHEN and *The Research Critique.* In *The anniversary book: A history of nursing in the west 1956-1992* (pp. 43-49). Boulder, CO: WIN.

Lindeman, C. A. (1992). Nursing research development. In *The anniversary book: A history of nursing in the West 1956-1992* (pp. 89-92). Boulder, CO: WIN.

McNeil, P. A. (2003). Foreword. In *Communicating Nursing Research, 36; WIN Assembly 11* (p. xix). Portland, OR: WIN.

McNeil, P. A. (2007). Foreword. In *Communicating Nursing Research, 40; WIN Assembly 15* (p. xxv). Portland, OR: WIN.

McNeil, P. A., & Lindeman, C. A. (in press). A history of the Western Institute of Nursing and its *Communicating Nursing Research* conferences. *Nursing Research.*

Mitchell, P. H. (2008). Knowledge that matters: Integrating research, practice, and education. In *Communicating Nursing Research, 41; WIN Assembly 16* (pp. 3-7). Portland, OR: WIN.

NEXus. (2016). The history of NEXus. Retrieved December 30, 2016 from http://winnexus.org/history.

Nyamathi, A. M. (2014). Going global: Past decade of nurse-led intervention research in developing countries. *Communicating Nursing Research, 47; WIN Assembly, 22* (pp. 17-26). Portland, OR: WIN.

Pepper, G. A. (2010). Bridges on the river why. In *Communicating Nursing Research, 43; WIN Assembly, 18* (pp. 45-58). Portland, OR: WIN.

Pine, L. A., & Burman, M. E. (2009, March, April). Wyoming Nurses Association dedicate this issue in the memory of Carol Macnee and Susan McCabe. *Wyoming Nurse, 22(1),* 1.

The Denver Channel. (2008, December 19). 2 UW professors die in highway 287 crash. Retrieved February 19, 2017 from http://www.thedenverchannel.com/news/2-uw-professors-die-in-highway-278-crash.

Voss, J. G. (2014). Innovations in nursing education in resource-constrained settings. In *Communicating Nursing Research, 47; WIN Assembly, 22* (pp. 27-35). Portland, OR: WIN.

Young, H. M. (2013). Nurses leading change, advancing health: Our campaign for action. Keynote Address in *Communicating Nursing Research, 46; WIN Assembly, 21* (pp. 3-6). Portland, OR: WIN.

Western Council on Higher Education for Nursing (WCHEN). (1957). *Charter of the Western Council on Higher Education for Nursing of the Western Interstate Commission for Higher Education.* Boulder, DO: WICHE. In P.P. Coulter (1963, July). *The winds of change* (Appendix c, pp. 63-66). Boulder, CO: WICHE. WIN archives, Portland, OR. Also in WIN (2007). *The anniversary book: 50 years of advancing nursing in the West 1957-2007* (pp. 27-36). Portland, OR: WIN.

Western Institute of Nursing (WIN). (1991, May 1-4). Fifth Annual WIN Assembly and 24th Annual Communicating Nursing Research Conference Program. WIN Archives, Portland, OR.

Western Institute of Nursing (WIN). (1992). *The anniversary book: A history of nursing in the West: 1956-1992.* Boulder, CO: WIN.

Western Institute of Nursing (WIN). (1993). *Communicating Nursing Research, 26; WIN Assembly, 1.* Boulder, CO: WIN.

Western Institute of Nursing (WIN). (1995). *Communicating Nursing Research, 28; WIN Assembly, 3.* Boulder, CO: WIN.

Western Institute of Nursing (WIN). (2000). *Communicating Nursing Research, 33; WIN Assembly, 8.* Portland, OR: WIN.

Western Institute of Nursing (WIN). (2001). *Communicating Nursing Research, 34; WIN Assembly, 9.* Portland, OR: WIN.

Western Institute of Nursing (WIN). (2002). *Communicating Nursing Research, 35; WIN Assembly, 10.* Portland, OR: WIN.

Western Institute of Nursing (WIN). (2003). *Communicating Nursing Research, 36; WIN Assembly, 11.* Portland, OR: WIN.

Western Institute of Nursing (WIN). (2004). *Communicating Nursing Research, 37; WIN Assembly, 12.* Portland, OR: WIN.

Western Institute of Nursing (WIN). (2005). *Communicating Nursing Research, 38; WIN Assembly, 13.* Portland, OR: WIN.

Western Institute of Nursing (WIN). (2006). *Communicating Nursing Research, 39; WIN Assembly, 14.* Portland, OR: WIN.

Western Institute of Nursing (WIN). (2007a). *Communicating Nursing Research, 40; WIN Assembly, 15.* Portland, OR: WIN.

Western Institute of Nursing (WIN). (2007b). *The anniversary book: 50 years of advancing nursing in the West 1957-2007.* Portland, OR: WIN.

Western Institute of Nursing (WIN). (2008). *Communicating Nursing Research, 41; WIN Assembly, 16.* Portland, OR: WIN.

Western Institute of Nursing (WIN). (2009). *Communicating Nursing Research, 42; WIN Assembly, 17.* Portland, OR: WIN.

Western Institute of Nursing (WIN). (2010). *Communicating Nursing Research, 43; WIN Assembly, 18.* Portland, OR: WIN.

Western Institute of Nursing (WIN). (2011a). *Communicating Nursing Research, 44; WIN Assembly, 19.* Portland, OR: WIN.

Western Institute of Nursing (WIN). (2011b, April 13). *WIN mission statement: Western Institute of Nursing strategic mission, vision, and goals.* Retrieved February 7, 2017 from https://www.winursing.org/about-win/win-mission-statement/.

Western Institute of Nursing (WIN). (2012). *Communicating Nursing Research, 45; WIN Assembly, 20.* Portland, OR: WIN.

Western Institute of Nursing (WIN). (2013). *Communicating Nursing Research, 46; WIN Assembly, 21.* Portland, OR: WIN.

Western Institute of Nursing (WIN). (2014). *Communicating Nursing Research, 47; WIN Assembly, 22.* Portland, OR: WIN.

Western Institute of Nursing (WIN). (2015). *Communicating Nursing Research, 48; WIN Assembly, 23.* Portland, OR: WIN.

Western Institute of Nursing (WIN). (2016a). *Communicating Nursing Research, 49; WIN Assembly, 24.* Portland, OR: WIN.

Western Institute of Nursing (WIN). (2016b). About WIN: History of WIN. Retrieved January 22, 2017 from https://www.winursing.org/about-win/.

Western Interstate Commission for Higher Education (WICHE). (2016). *About WICHE.* Boulder, CO: WICHE. Retrieved July 14, 2016 from http://www.wiche.edu/about.

Young, H. M., Bakewell-Sachs, S., & Sarna, L. (in press). Nursing practice, research, and education in the West: The best is yet to come. *Nursing Research.*

Chapter Six

Communicating Nursing Research:
50 YEARS AND BEYOND

Chapter Six
Communicating Nursing Research:
50 YEARS AND BEYOND
Elaine S. Marshall & Barbara Gaines

Somewhere in the West, a brisk breeze is always blowing – a current which may unpredictably become a whirlwind, sweeping before it outgrown traditions and practices and creating space for innovation, experimentation, and progress. The West is changing – on the move – and nursing is changing and moving with it (Coulter, 1963, p. 1).

Pearl Parvin Coulter titled her treatise *The Winds of Change* in 1963. Even then, her concepts of "outgrown tradition" versus "space for innovation, experimentation, and progress" foretold the philosophy that would be the continuing voice of nursing in the West: collaboration in education, practice, research, and contribution to disciplinary growth. While the "winds" might be interpreted at first glance as the random and unpredictable Western tumbleweed, implicit in Coulter's description is the focused intention that changes in nursing in the West would respect its roots while growing to its desired future. The Preface to the *Anniversary Book* of the celebration of 50 years of the Western Institute of Nursing (WIN) acknowledges the planning committee's "resolute belief" that this conference provided both the "joyous opportunity to look back at the proud accomplishments . . . and a conference program that helps the organization set an agenda for the next 50!" (WIN, 2007, p. v.)

The Early Vision
Nursing research in the West grew out of a commitment of its early nurse educators associated with the Western Interstate Commission for Higher Education (WICHE) to improve nursing education and practice. The understanding that collaboration and sharing resources were the best means for nurses in this large and diverse geographic region to improve patient care through education and research was based on a strong knowledge foundation that guided the work of these leaders through its history (Abbott, 2004).

Within five years of the inception of WICHE in 1951, its leaders recognized the need to foster graduate education in nursing and convened a leadership group to address that need. A flurry of activity followed. Within the year, there was a major survey of nursing education programs, a meeting of 100 representatives of nursing education and practice to launch program directions, the appointment of the original Committee of Seven that would propose what eventually became WCHEN and plant the seeds of what would become the "research conference." The commitment to work together in a philosophy of shared ideas and resources as the way forward for professional nursing in the West was firmly in place. All that was needed was a funding source and professional staff to make the plans a reality. A grant from the W. K. Kellogg Foundation and the hiring of Jo Eleanor Elliott provided the welcome answers (Abbott, 2004; WIN, 1992, p. 9; WIN, 2007, p. 39).

Early nursing leaders in the West understood that the highest quality nursing education to provide the best patient care was dependent on solid disciplinary growth through research. Vision was required. There were "only a half dozen programs preparing nurses for leadership positions in nursing education; essentially no body of nursing research; and around 10 nurses with doctoral degrees and . . . these were in disciplines other than nursing" (McNeil & Lindeman, in press). Research needed to be integral to the entire work of the discipline, not an additional activity reserved for an elite few. Early attention was focused on developing research skills and advancing graduate education for nursing faculty in the region.

Classic Works and Beyond from the *Communicating Nursing Research Conference:* Contributions to the Discipline

A history of any professional enterprise, such as a conference, needs to respond to more than its simple chronology. There is always the essential question of "so what?" What do we learn from its history of the enduring value of the *Communicating Nursing Research* conference? What does it contribute to the discipline?

One might easily argue that the vision, leadership, and engagement alone proved enough to inspire the advancement of the values of research to build the science, the innovation to promote new ways of thinking and practice, and participation in the national and international scene as both model and participant to improve health care. But a journey through a small, select group of presentations from the *Communicating Nursing Research* conference offers some examples of profound contributions that came from the conference.

Three presentations, "Classic Work of Our Members" (WIN, 2007, p. 91), highlight the early work of pioneers as models for consideration, with the acknowledgement that they are only representatives of some of the best of the work from the conference. There are dozens of other examples with similar influence. These models were reprinted in *the Anniversary Book: 50 Years of Advancing Nursing in the West* in 2007 (WIN, 2007, pp. 91-125), and continue to be considered classics. They bear revisiting today: *The Research Critique: Nature, Function, and Art* by Madeleine Leininger in 1968, *Discipline of Nursing: Structure and Relationship to Practice* by Sue Donaldson and Dorothy Crowley in 1977, and *Advancing Nursing Science: Qualitative Approaches* by Jeanne Quint Benoliel in 1984. These became classics in the discipline for their decade. Today, each WIN member might ask, what are the classics of my own time at WIN?

Leininger and The Research Critique. The question of the role of critique in developing a quality research conference in the West was raised at the WCHEN regional conference in 1958 by one who is best known at the same conference for his suggestion that nurses should not engage in independent research (WCHEN, 1958; 1960, pp. 77-79). The issue of the value of critique to the research enterprise in the West did not go away and has remained a concern for many subsequent conference planning committees.

In her presentation ten years later at the first *Communicating Nursing Researc* conference, Leininger found the issue of critique to be relevant and vexing. As she argued the difference between review and critique, she cited two examples to make her point. One was a 1966 editorial in *Nursing Research* (Editorial, 1966), that she interpreted, "Essentially, the function of the research critique is to help the researcher refine his research study or to develop a better study in the future" (Leininger, 1968, p. 95). The second reference was to Henry James: "The practice of 'reviewing' . . . in general has nothing in common with the art of criticism" (James, 1893). As she moved forward her argument for "critique" rather "review," Leininger elaborated the elements and collaborative process necessary to do good critique. Batey (1968, p. v) shared that Leininger's presentation sent the first critiquers scurrying to revise their presentations to meet her challenging assertions. Her presentation set the stage for what would become an integral process to the conference. And while the purposes of critique as originally envisioned would change as the conference grew and changed through activities such as symposia, research clinics, discussions, and poster sessions (McNeil & Lindeman, in press), the concept of collaborative exchange to improve the knowledge base for the discipline and the expectation of the highest quality were institutionalized. Discussants, as a formal response to research presented, have even been reintroduced in the anniversary conference in 2017 (personal communication, P. McNeil, December 2016).

Donaldson and Crowley on a Discipline for Nursing. The second paper selected as a classic was that by Donaldson and Crowley (1977) that promulgated the idea that a discipline has boundaries. This notion confronted what authors saw as a fragmented approach to a body of knowledge that had held nursing back in its attempts to grow as a discipline within the confines of higher education. It also provoked nurses to change practice from task rituals to full acceptance as a knowledge-based profession. Donaldson and Crowley cited three themes with many examples from available nursing literature that have consistently guided nurse scholars since the time of Nightingale. The themes were the following:

1. Concern with principles and laws that govern life processes, well-being, and optimum functioning of human beings sick or well . . .
2. Concern with the pattern of human behavior in interaction with the environment in critical life situations . . .
3. Concern with processes by which positive changes in health status are affected... (Donaldson & Crowley, 1977, pp. 105-106)

The influence of Donaldson and Crowley is visible in the following concepts of the definition of nursing by the American Nurses Association in 2017: "protection, promotion, and optimization of health and abilities" and "diagnosis and treatment of human responses" (ANA, 2017).

Donaldson and Crowley also presented arguments to promote the disciplinary, scientific, and practical concerns of nursing with examples of the importance of each. Citing Schwab (1964), they argued for both the "substantive structure . . . conceptualization . . . based on their fit with the perspective of the discipline" and for the "syntactical structure . . . research methodologies and criteria used to justify the acceptance of truth of statements within the discipline" (p. 115).

Benoliel and the Qualitative Paradigm. In 1984, the question of the necessary spectrum of methods useful to nurse researchers rose to the forefront. Jeanne Benoliel tackled the question, and raised the discussion to the concept of the syntactical structure of the discipline noted earlier by Donaldson and Crowley. Benoliel argued for an alternative paradigm, one based on "some general beliefs about the nature of human beings and their individual and social relationship" and made the case for truth in the paradigm with the comment, "In this perspective on knowledge, truth is not absolute but exists in multiple forms" (pp. 121-122). Benoliel extended her argument to consider the qualitative paradigm and issues of validity, theoretical and methodological perspectives, and trying out the research process. She concluded her argument:

Qualitative inquiry can be used to expand knowledge about human experience at many levels of existence . . . It is an orientation toward the production of knowledge based on a belief that the central activity of science is the use of various patterns of reasoning, identified by Suppe (1977, p. 657) as "different systems of rules of the scientific game" (Benoliel, 1984, p. 125).

Evolving Classics as New Questions Expand the Science

The contributions of these three papers to the definition and evaluation of knowledge of the discipline allowed nurse researchers in the West to explore new questions that continued to advance both the science and the practice of nursing. This statement is generously supported by the "predictions and promises" of leading researchers quoted within this chapter.

One example of the continuing extension of the knowledge base to new questions is the presentation by Linda Lange at the Sixth annual *WIN Assembly* in 1992, *Using Clinical Data to Enhance Nursing Outcomes.* Lange addressed the emerging relationship between nursing and the broader conception of health care/services research and health informatics. Lange framed her discussion of minimum data sets within the topic of clinical data used by nurses to improve nursing outcomes. She explained a major premise guiding her understanding:

By documenting clinical data and information, nurses gain the additional ability to create knowledge from the experiences of other nurses, and to understand how actions and outcomes are related to over the entire course of a patient's illness. The circle is closed when nurses are able to use the documented record of past experience to make clinical decisions about patients presently assigned to their care (Lange, 1992, p. 3).

Like the Lange exposition of nursing as integral to the broader area of health care/services research, numerous examples of research challenging the old boundaries of the discipline of nursing can be found in the State of the Science papers, podium presentations, and poster sessions through the years at the *Communicating Nursing Research* conference. The 50th conference will not be an exception.

In their State of the Science session of 2017, Linda Sarna, Heather Young, and Susan Bakewell-Sachs (WIN, 2017) remind that the 50th anniversary conference year also marks 30 years of the National Institute of Nursing Research and the 15-year anniversary of the Council of the Advancement of Nursing Science. The authors address issues of importance to nursing education, nursing practice, and the broader field of health care. They elaborate on the concerns about research for the continued growth of the discipline. They note especially the lack of Ph.D. prepared researchers and faculty prepared to address a wide variety of topics from "omics" to "big data" requiring a nursing lens to improve the health care of individuals, families, and society in a cost efficient manner. The authors conclude by challenging nurses to use their collaborative past to create a collective future. They propose:

As we face the increasing demands in a time of fewer resources, collaboration across our region and beyond will assure that we continue to innovate and deliver excellence in nursing practice, research, and education. The call has never been louder, our collective strength has never been as impressive, and our responsibility is ever greater (Young, Bakewell-Sachs, & Sarna, in press, p. 18).

The Continuing Success of the *Communicating Nursing Research* Conference
The *Communicating Nursing Research* conference has continued to grow in participation, stature, and excellence for 50 years. Various traditions have grown over the years, but consistency has continued. Chief among the factors of success has been consistent excellent executive leadership. In its 60 years, WIN has had four executive directors: Jo Eleanor Elliott, Sally Ruybal, Jeanne Kearns, and Paula McNeil. Three of these leaders have each served the organization for at least 20 years. All have served with distinction, facing limited resources; continuing challenges for innovation, collaboration, communication, and coordination among changing structures, different styles of governing boards, and collaborative organizations; ever-growing demands for new programs; and positive representation of the organization at national and international levels. Beyond growing demands on a broad range of expectations, each has produced an outstanding annual conference for *Communicating Nursing Research*.

The conference has continued to build on important traditions that reach beyond simple research dissemination. Following are some examples:

Each session follows a theme based on timely issues, events, and/or policies.
Each session features an exemplary Keynote Address.
Each session offers innovative State of the Science papers.
Each session rewards its best with honors that extend the mission of the conference:
    The Distinguished Research Lectureship
    The Carol Lindeman New Researcher Award
    The Jo Eleanor Elliott Leadership Award
    The Anna M. Shannon Mentorship Award
    The Patsy A. Perry Physiologic Nursing Research Award
    The Ann M. Voda American Indian/Alaska Native/First Nation Conference Award
    The John A. Hartford Foundation/WIN Geriatric Nursing Education and
        Research Awards
    Induction into the Western Academy of Nurses
    Bestowal of Emeriti Status.
Each session features updates on federal and other funding opportunities.
Each session publishes major addresses and abstracts of presentations in one of the most respected volumes of proceedings.
Each session features a panel or presentation from the Western Academy of Nurses.
Each session features opportunities for research development in special sessions or by the Research Information Exchange.
Each session features opportunities for networking, friendships, and fun.

The conference has grown in reputation as a gathering place for professional networking and friendship. The personal reflections of Elizabeth Nichols 25 years ago "On Spider Webs and Snowflakes," describe sentiments that continue today:

How do networks develop? Are they the fruit of hard work and persistence, much like the spider web spanning a window corner, or are they the result of the random action of nature like the snowflake falling through the winter air? Networks, like both snowflakes and spider webs have a center

127

- the individual nurse researcher. The branches of the network spread out in response to the particular needs or interests of the researcher . . .

Networks spawn new ideas, new liaisons, new projects, and new friends. Thus it is with WSRN. Networks also support and strengthen old relationships and bring new dimensions into these relationships.

I have grown up with WSRN. It has always been there, and has, for me provided an opportunity and a support structure for my professional and personal growth . . .

[My first WSRN conference] was an excursion into the land of the giants. The giants of nursing research and nursing leadership (Nichols, 1992, p. 131).

Communicating Nursing Research: By the Numbers

A review of the data across the history of the conference reveals a total of 4,487 presenters at the podium (named on podium or symposia). Among these, 2,866 have presented once, 1,621 presented two or more times, more than 160 people were named on podium or symposia presentations at least 10 times, and 40 people have presented 20 or more times. Table 6-1 lists WIN members who were represented more than 40 times in the history of the conference, listed in order of the number of their presentations.

Most of the people on this list have extended mentorship to include novice researchers on symposia they have led, have distinguished themselves nationally and internationally, and they have shown by their participation in the *Communicating Nursing Research* conference extraordinary commitment to nursing research in the West. The list is not exhaustive of the outstanding researchers of our time, but their names represent the best of every scholar committed to the advancement of nursing knowledge to improve practice, education, and policy.

Table 6-1. Researchers Listed on at Least 40 Lectures, Podium, or Symposia Presentations at the *Communicating Nursing Research* Conference In Order of Number of Times Presenting

Nancy F. Woods	Monica Jarrett
Ellen S. Mitchell	Joan Shaver
Clarann Weinert	Souraya Sidani
Martha J. Lentz	Lynn C. Callister
Heather M. Young	Nancy E. Donaldson
Deborah Koniak-Griffin	Ada S. Hinshaw
Joyce A. Verran	Adeline M. Nyamathi
Barbara Mandleco	Terry Badger
Karen G. Schepp	Kathryn A. Lee
Paula Meek	Robert L. Burr
Lauren Clark	Ramona Mercer
Sandra Ferketich	Marcia Killien
Margaret Heitkemper	Marie-Annette Brown
Ginette Pepper	Carrie J. Merkle
	Marie Lobo

Seven Scholars. In the spirit of WIN's two distinguished Committees of Seven, fifty years is celebrated by a glimpse at the seven most prolific speakers at the *Communicating Nursing Research* conference:

Nancy Woods has presented far and above any presenter at the conference. She is Dean Emerita, Professor, and Co-Director of the de Tornyay Center for Healthy Aging at the University of Washington. She graduated from the University of Wisconsin Eau Claire, earned the master's degree from the University of Washington, and completed the Ph.D. at the University of North Carolina Chapel Hill. She received the Pathfinder Award from the Friends of the National Institute for Nursing Research and was elected to the Institute of Medicine (Woods, 2017). Her name has appeared on the Conference program nearly 100 times, including numerous symposia, Keynote Address, Distinguished Research Lecture, State of the Science paper, and Western Academy of Nursing panel. Following are her own words from the University of Washington website:

> I have led a sustained program of research in the field of women's health. With collaborators from nursing and other fields, I have contributed to an improved understanding of women's experiences of menstrual cycle symptoms as well as the menopausal transition, investigating endocrine, social, personal, and genetic factors influencing symptoms and women's approaches to symptom management. In 1989, Dr. Joan Shaver and I, in collaboration with other colleagues, established the first NIH-funded Center for Women's Health Research . . . Dr. Ellen Mitchell and I established the Seattle Midlife Women's Health Study . . . involving over 500 women, some of whom we studied for up to 25 years (Woods, 2017).

Ellen Sullivan Mitchell completed the Ph.D. from the University of Washington. She was a nurse practitioner specializing in adult primary care. She is now retired associate professor from the University of Washington, and continues her research related to menopausal transition (Mitchell, 2017). She was involved for years in longitudinal research projects on women's health with Nancy Woods at the University of Washington, including the Seattle Midlife Women's Health Study (Woods, 2017). She was the second most frequent presenter in 50 years at the *Communicating Nursing Research* conference, usually in symposia on women's health projects, and she appeared on a Western Academy of Nurses panel.

Clarann Weinert graduated from College of Mount St. Joseph on the Ohio, earned master's degrees from The Ohio State University and the University of Washington, and the Ph.D. from the University of Washington. She is a Sister of Charity of Cincinnati. She is now Professor Emerita from Montana State University. She is best known for a career of more than 25 years devoted to research in areas of rural health and social support (see Weinert, 2011). At WIN, besides many research presentations, she has been a Distinguished Research Lecturer, presented two State of the Science papers, and has appeared on a Western Academy of Nurses panel.

Martha J. Lentz is a Research Professor Emerita at the University of Washington. She completed her undergraduate work at Wayne State University in Detroit Michigan. She obtained her Ph.D. as part of the first class at the University of Washington. It was through encouragement by mentors during her doctoral program that she began her first research presentations at WIN. Her primary research area is sleep and biological rhythms in interaction with symptoms in chronic health conditions. Strong methodological and statistical skills led her to participate in a wide range of research studies. She has been honored by WIN with the Distinguished Research Lecture, State of the Science paper, has presented on a Western Academy of Nurses panel, and continues to present her research at the *Communicating Nursing Research* conference.

Heather M. Young is Associate Vice Chancellor for Nursing, Dean, and Professor of the Betty Irene Moore School of Nursing at University of California Davis (UC Davis). She graduated from UC Davis in Dietetics and Southern Oregon State College in nursing. She earned the M.S. and the Ph.D. degrees at the University of Washington. Her expertise is gerontological nursing and rural health care. She "researches healthy aging with a particular focus on the interface between individuals and family as well as formal health care systems." She currently leads a large study to improve health for individuals with diabetes, funded by the Patient-Centered Outcomes Research Institute (Young, 2017). She also works on the national Strategic Advisory Committee of the Robert Wood Johnson Foundation and the California Action Coalition executive committee to implement the 2011 Institute of Medicine report on *The Future of Nursing*. At the *Communicating Nursing Research* conference, she has been a Keynote speaker, State of the Science presenter, and served on a panel of the Western Academy of Nurses.

Deborah Koniak-Griffin is a Professor and Associate Dean of the Office of Diversity, Equity, and Inclusion at the University of California Los Angeles. Her research, funded by the National Institutes of Health (NIH), spans over twenty years on "the development and evaluation of health promotion/disease prevention interventions to eliminate health disparities in vulnerable populations of youth and adult women" (Koniak-Griffin, 2017). She also collaborates as the principle investigator on a Fogarty International Training Grant with a school of nursing in Changsha, China. She has been the Distinguished Research Lecturer, State of the Science speaker, and panelist with the Western Academy of Nurses at the *Communicating Nursing Research* conference.

Joyce A. Verran has devoted more than 25 years to funded research in areas of nursing care delivery systems. Her research has spanned acute care environments, complexity of care in ambulatory settings, and nursing practice models in rural communities. She graduated from Los Angeles USC Medical Center, and earned the B.S.N., M.S., and Ph.D. from the University of Arizona (Verran, 2017), where she spent much of her career. She was a Visiting Professor at the University of Colorado Denver. She was also honored by WIN with the Distinguished Research Lectureship, State of the Science presentation, and Western Academy of Nurses panel.

One indicator of commitment is the willingness to critique, discuss, or moderate sessions. Table 6-2 lists scholars who have most frequently served, in order of number of times they acted as moderators and discussants.

Another example of the continuing outstanding leadership in the West is the number of Living Legends of the American Academy of Nursing with roots in in WIN. Many of the following have appeared as key figures in the history of WIN: Faye Abdellah, Kathryn Barnard, Patricia Benner, Jeanne Benoliel, Linda Bolton, Marie Cowan, Anne Davis, Rheba de Tornyay, Marylin Dodd, Kathleen Dracup, Barbara Durand, Loretta Ford, Colleen Goode, Susan Gortner, Ada Sue Hinshaw, Marlene Kramer, Madeleine Leininger, Afaf Meleis, Ramona Mercer, Jessie Scott, Gladys Sorensen, Jean Watson, and Betty Williams (see Living Legends, 2016).

Table 6-2 Critiquers, Discussants, Moderators for Podium Sessions At the *Communicating Nursing Research* Conference Listed in Order of Frequency of Service	
Critique	**Moderator**
Janelle Krueger	Tina DeLapp
Pamela Brink	Marie Driever
Marlene Kramer	Terry Badger
Dorothy Martin	Maureen O'Malley
Frank McLaughlin	Marcia Killien
	Martha Lentz
Discussant	Kathleen Chafey
Ann Davis	Jay Shen
Lulu Hassenplug	Donna Velasquez
Janelle Krueger	Carol Ashton
Ruth Ludemann	Carrie Jo Braden
Jean Lum	Patricia Butterfield
	Beverly Hoeffer

Young, Bakewell-Sachs, and Sarna (in press) further highlighted Western nursing leaders in research in the country who merit some note. They listed WIN members, Ada Sue Hinshaw and Nancy Woods who were at the table at the development of the National Institute of Nursing Research (NINR); Betty Chang and Marie Cowan as members of the first Study Section at NINR; and Friends of NINR Pathfinder Award recipients from the West, Margaret Heitkemper, Deborah Koniak-Griffin, Carol Landis, Pamela Mitchell, Ida (Ki) Moore, Linda Phillips, [and Nancy Woods] (Young, et. al., in press). Table 6-3 lists WIN members inducted into the Sigma Theta Tau International Nurse Researcher Hall of Fame (see STTI, 2017).

Table 6-3 Researchers with Ties to WIN and the West Inducted into the Sigma Theta Tau International Nurse Researcher Hall of Fame	
Kathryn Barnard	Merle Mishel
Marylin Dodd	Pamela Mitchell
Cynthia Dougherty	Ida (Ki) Moore
Betty Farrell	Janice Morse
Margaret Heitkemper	Adeline Nyamathi
William Holzemer	Linda Sarna
Deborah Koniak-Griffin	Joan Shaver
Kathryn Lee	Clarann Weinert
Usha Menon	Nancy Woods
Christine Miaskowski	

What's in a Name?

Among the first ten titles of the 50 *Communicating Nursing Research* conferences, only two titles contained a colon (20% colons). However, among the last 10 titles, only two titles did not contain a colon (80% colons). This has been a more trivial, but actual point of discussion in professional publication. A few scholars have studied the influence of title structure on research dissemination. Dillon (1981, p. 879) analyzed titles of 30 "prominent journals in psychology, education, and literary criticism" to find that the presence of a colon in the title increased "publishability, productivity, complexity of thought, distinction of endeavor, and progress of the enterprise." Huggett (2011) graphed titles in the journal *Cell* showing that titles with a comma or colon were more likely to be cited. Fox and Burns (2015) noted that papers with subtitles (which might assume a colon) were less likely to be rejected by editors for a different specific scientific journal.

On a similar note, the words that most often followed the colon in the conference title were some version of "research, practice, and education." These words did not appear in a title of the *Communicating Nursing Research* conference until 1994, then in 1996, and not again until 2005. But in the last ten years, correlating with the high number of colons, six of the ten titles contain the words "research, practice, and education" in some order. This provokes the question of what is the need for the more recent annual reminder of the mission of education, practice, and research? Other word selections seem to reflect favorite trends in jargon of the time. Examples include the following: "the image of nursing research" in 1983, as nursing and women were struggling for credibility and social power; "quality" in 1998 and 2004 as issues of quality and safety were highlighted by IOM reports; "health disparities" in 2002 at the time when this concept became common in health care discussions; "innovation" in 1995, 2005, 2012, 2016 as it becomes a growing theme. Are conference titles and topics leading to set new standards or following trends? How can nurses of the West assure advancement toward a visionary future, to move beyond reflecting current or past initiatives and/or issues?

Looking Back at Predictions and Promises

Twenty-five years ago, at the silver anniversary of the *Communicating Nursing Research* conference, several great minds of the West offered their observations and recorded their predictions:

Mary Jane Ward, member of the WICHE/WCHEN staff from 1975 to 1979 observed (1992, p. 99):

It would be hard, if not impossible, to evaluate the impact of WIN/ WCHEN and WSRN on nursing research not only in the West but in other areas of the world as well. The nursing research projects conducted under their leadership and the nurses introduced to the need for and excitement of conducting research have greatly influenced patient care, the profession, and nursing education

Betty Mitsunaga, the first Chair of the Research Steering Committee for the conference under WSRN, predicted the following (1992, p. 86-87):

The directions that nursing research will take in the future will be influenced by a number of factors, including the priorities of funding agencies, the trendiness of certain problem areas, research programs that continue to evolve, new clinical nursing problems that emerge . . . changes in the delivery of health care, development of new technology, and so on. There is no doubt that research by nurses will be more widely recognized for the contributions made to knowledge about health and health care . . .

Increased . . . attention needs to be directed to certain issues . . . research that is focused on or inclusive of ethnic minority populations. Although the National Institutes of Health have given impetus to inclusion of minorities as research subjects, simple inclusion is not sufficient. Cultural sensitivity is a major consideration in relation of appropriate comparison groups; instrument development; use of existing instruments; data-gathering procedures; and data analysis and interpretation . . .

To what extent have minority populations been a focus or explicitly included in research reported at the WIN/WSRN conference? . . .

Another issue which needs increased attention is theory development . . . in the case of qualitative research, development of theory based on outcomes of a single study may be premature. On the other hand, how many descriptions of a phenomenon are needed to develop a theory? . . . In order to further develop nursing science, fragments of knowledge need to be conceptually organized and the linkages tested for fuller understanding of phenomena.

Finally, the effort to link research to practice is a continuing goal. Visible progress has been made, certainly, but much of nursing practice remains to be studied and research findings incorporated into practice . . .

If progress in nursing research is made in the next 25 years at the same rate as the past 25 years, the above issues will be resolved before 2017 and new issues which challenge us will be topics of the WIN/WSRN conference that year. What will they be?

May Rawlinson predicted that "integrated computer communications" might provide new means for people to communicate, citing and envisioning "an imaginary conference room where teams of people will be brought together by means of their computers from all over the world to collaborate on a given project" (Chilles, 1991; Rawlinson, 1992, p. 113). Ginette Pepper (1992) also predicted electronic books and journals.

Regarding research in the practice setting, Carolyn Murdaugh (1992, p. 121) predicted with hope the growth of clinical nurse research positions, closer collaboration between clinical agencies and universities in planning clinical learning activities for undergraduate and graduate students to facilitate role models for "science based practice," and collaboration between nursing and other disciplines to facilitate "science-based practice" and "financial viability" of clinical research departments. Pepper (1992, p. 142) confirmed those hopeful predictions and mused on whether nursing research might be "predominantly in the service setting," whether the focus in the clinical setting might be research generation or research utilization, and noted that new and creative funding sources must be developed. She asked, "Will clinically-based research activities continue to thrive in the U. S., and specifically in the West? What should be the relationship between clinical and academic nursing research? And what should be the focus of clinically-based nursing research?"

Virginia Tilden (1992, pp 136-139) predicted the following for our time:

With great confidence, I predict that nursing research will continue to achieve expanded visibility in both the federal and private funding sectors, that more findings from nursing research will make the evening news, and that nurse researchers increasingly will collaborate with other health disciplines in solving the Nation's health problems.

Twenty-five years ago, Tilden's further predictions included the following: (1) Move of the (then) National Center for Nursing Research to become the National Institute for Nursing Research, (2) A growth in federally funded post-doctoral career development awards, (3) An increase in sophistication of institutional processes to support stellar proposals that will attract funding to nurse researchers even in times of reduced funding levels, (4) Increased collaboration among health care disciplines in research with associated "recognition and respect for the research training of nurse investigators," (5) Leadership among nurse researchers in the growing focus on attention to the health of women, minorities, and the underserved (Tilden, 1992, pp. 137-138).

Tilden (1992, p. 139) boldly concluded:

Twenty-five years from now, WSRN will celebrate its 50th anniversary. The year will be 2017. The National Institute of Nursing Research . . . will be funded equally with medicine and dentistry. The vast majority of NIH funded research will be collaborative between nursing, medicine, and at least one other appropriate discipline . . . The majority of nurse investigators will have postdoctoral research training and will have ongoing programs of research in a focused area where each study informs the next. Through its support of nurse researchers in the West and its role in shaping nursing's national research agenda, WSRN will have helped bring these dreams to reality.

The Golden Anniversary and Ahead
    The conference has set the standard for any forum to advance the science of nursing in order to improve health throughout the country and the world. In the past 50 years, one can only wonder:

• How many studies were born from ideas during presentations, lunch and reception conversations, and personal mentoring consultations that happened at the conference?
• How many studies were eventually funded by consultation with federal officers who regularly attended the conference?
• How many endowed chairs or distinguished professorships were filled from personal and professional connections at the conference?
• In how many ways was health care improved by the works of participants of the conference?

Susan Gortner (1992, p. 64) noted, ". . . the style and ambiance of the WICHE [WSRN] research conferences became a model for other regional and national nursing research conferences." Gortner (1992, p. 64) also noted the special value in the attendance of officers of Federal nursing research programs "to discuss proposals with prospective applicants and to provide information on Federal grant and fellowship programs. The annual research conferences became an increasingly important forum for information exchange between academic and Federal colleagues" (Gortner, 1992, p. 64).

Leininger noted (1992, p. 45):

. . . . Many outstanding nurse research methodologists and theorists came from the WCHEN/WIN research conferences. These organizational structures and prevailing research ethos provided the "cultural glue" to support many nurse leaders to engage in quality research investigations. WCHEN as the first cultural structure, encouraged nurses to share ideas with each other and to value nursing research as essential for the discipline of nursing. It was this nursing culture that helped establish norms to maintain not only nursing research, but also quality nursing education and client nursing services in the West.

Though her reflections were 25 years ago, the memories of Benoliel (1992, p. 128-129) live even today:

It is impressive how far we have come from the early days of being defensive about nurses' rights to do research to the current involvement in sophisticated multidisciplinary investigations and the politics of influencing the direction of health care delivery . . . These conferences were the settings in which we gained experience in presenting research, met people whose work we admired, sought counsel from the "feds," talked with journal editors about how to get published, participated in networks with people having similar interests, and offered guidance to others . . .

The conferences served as birthing sites for the creating of new enterprises [such as the *Western Journal of Nursing Research*] . . . and recruiting sites for deans in search of new faculty and for faculty in search of new positions.

Participation in these conferences also was a very human experience in which we shared the latest gossip, learned a lot about the realities of research and the complexities of people, and watched the developing careers of future leaders, e. g., Ada Sue Hinshaw, Kathy Barnard, Merle Mishel, Jane Norbeck, Barbara Walike, Nancy Woods, Patricia Benner, and many others. Participation in the conferences brought much fun and laughter when groups got together after a hard day's work . . . for food, drink, and relaxation . . .

Membership in the group also brought its moments of poignancy [as when we lost beloved members] . . . The nursing community has lost many of the early pioneers whose dreams made these conferences a reality. In a singular way the conferences are a living memorial to the vision and commitment of these far-sighted nurses.

On to the Future
Young and colleagues pointed to several nursing research needs of the future in the West and some initiatives to improve health. Examples include areas of focus in symptom science and symptom management, health promotion, health disparities, biobehavioral interventions, health informatics, various populations including rural communities, as well as specific issues and responses in nursing practice and education. They also made recommendations that bear striking similarity to WCHEN initiatives 50 years ago:

1. Establish WIN as a clearing house of best practices for addressing major health conditions and health promotion behaviors and health care organizational policies to optimize RN and APRN practice.
2. Launch a policy-focused effort within WIN for advocacy in health and health profession policy including workforce issues in the Western United States.
3. Organize results-focused forums for members to clarify problems, set priorities for addressing the problems, and collaborate to take actions to advance nursing practice, education, research, and policy in the Western United States to improve health and health care outcomes.
4. Identify three top priorities for each mission of practice, education, research, and policy to galvanize coordinated efforts for maximum effort and impact (Young, et al., in press).

One important element implied in the recommendations is the perennial challenge for WIN in financing its activities. Early leaders and current leaders were, and are, creative in developing resources to advance its mission. Continued collaboration, generous efforts and support, and innovation in development will continue to be important among the members of WIN to advance its work.

On the occasion of the 25th anniversary of the National Institute of Nursing Research at NIH in 2010, Patricia Grady made observations that may apply to WIN, the *Communicating Nursing Research* conference, and nursing in the West:

At no time has the nursing profession been transformed more dramatically than in the past thirty years. Behind that revolution, literally millions of nurses have constituted a team of committed actors: clinicians, professional nursing organizations, [and] schools of nursing . . . moved it beyond procedure to promise, beyond implementation to innovation, and into main stream science . . .

Over the years, nursing science directed at critical health outcomes has grown and developed a sophistication that is enabling our profession to translate scientific research and data into policy that helps shape the nation's healthcare system . . . Twenty-five years ago, only a small number of nurse researchers in the United States could claim advanced degrees in science. Today, there is an entire sector of the nursing profession populated with highly trained, innovative nurse scientists. Their growing body of work, often in tandem with other scientific disciplines, has altered the way Americans approach many health care issues . . .

Policies, informed and shaped by the research data of nurse scientists, have shortened hospital stays, decreased patient complications, increased patient satisfaction, and eased the transition to home care . . .

As the current debate over health care reform continues, nursing science, as it has in the past, will be at the forefront of designing programs that promote wellness, prevention, and not coincidentally, lower health care costs. The story of the NINR recounts the development and use of science to form new constructs of nursing practice—from observation to translation, from nursing care to nursing science, from procedure to practice to policy . . .

A tribute goes also to the millions of practicing nurses who support the ideas research entails and incorporate new science into their practices. Nurse scientists will always be a key wellspring of the information required so that evidence-based practice and policy can prevail and ensure the delivery of high-quality health care. I am confident that a continuing flow of fresh ideas and innovative science from nurse investigators will help reform and transform the American health care system in the twenty-first century (Grady, 2010, pp. v-viii).

Coulter's concept of the *Winds of Change* continues to describe the steady growth of vision, commitment, innovation, and advancement of better health care through nursing education, practice, and research. The story of the *Communicating Nursing Research* conference is a story of thousands of people who continue as pioneers in the West, lending their influence across the country and the world. It is unfortunate that space does not allow exploration of each individual life path. History needs to ask them about their inspirations, their failures, and their successes. We also need to know how they might assess the state of the discipline, how their work fits within the science, and its needs and ventures into the future. On to the next 50 years!

References

Abbott, F. C. (2004). *A history of the Western Interstate Commission for Higher Education: The first 40 years.* Boulder, CO: WICHE. See Note 1-D.

American Nurses Association (ANA). What is nursing? Retrieved February 19, 2017 from http://www.nursingworld.org/EspeciallyForYou/What-is-Nursing.

Batey, M. V. (Ed.) (1968). *Communicating Nursing Research, 1.* Boulder, CO: WCHEN.

Benoliel, J. Q. (1984). Advancing nursing science: Qualitative approaches. In *Communicating Nursing Research, 17.* Boulder, CO: WCHEN. Reprinted in WIN (2007) *The anniversary book: 50 years of advancing nursing in the West* (pp. 119-125). Portland, OR: WIN.

Benoliel, J. Q. (1992). The changing climate of WSRN conferences. In *The anniversary book: A history of nursing in the West 1956-1992* (pp. 125-129). Boulder, CO: WIN.

Chiles, J. R. (1992). Goodbye telephone, hello to new communications age. *Smithsonian, 22(11),* 46-56.

Coulter, P. P. (1963, July). *The winds of change: Progress report of regional cooperation in collegiate nursing education in the West.* Boulder, CO: WICHE. WIN archives, Portland, OR.

Dillon, J. T. (1981). The emergence of the colon: An empirical correlate of scholarship. *American Psychologist, 36(8),* 879-884.

Donaldson, S. K., & Crowley, D. M. (1977). Discipline of nursing: Structure and relationship to practice. In *Communicating Nursing Research, 10.* Boulder, CO: WCHEN. Reprinted in WIN (2007) *The anniversary book: 50 years of advancing nursing in the West* (pp. 105-118). Portland, OR: WIN.

Editorial. (1966). The research critique. *Nursing Research, 15(3),* 195.

Fox, C. W., & Burns, C. S. (2015). The relationship between manuscript title structure and success: Editorial decisions and citation performance for an ecological journal. *Ecology & Evolution, 5(10),* 1970-1980.

Gortner, S. R. (1992). The federal role. In *The anniversary book: A history of nursing in the West 1956-1992* (pp. 63-67). Boulder, CO: WIN.

Grady, P. A. (2010). Preface in P. L. Canelon, *NINR: Bringing science to life* (pp. v-viii). Bethesda, MD: NINR of NIH.

Huggett, S. (2011, September). Heading for success: Or how not to title your paper. *Research Trends, 24.* Retrieved February 8, 2017 from https://www. researchtrends.com/issue24-september-2011/heading-for-success-or-how-not-to-title-your-paper/.

James, H. (1893). Quotation from *Criticism.* In J. Bartlett (E. M. Beck, Ed.) (1980) *Bartlett's familiar quotations* (p. 653). Boston: Little, Brown, & Co.

Koniak-Griffin, D. (2017). Deborah Koniak-Griffin. Retrieved February 18, 2017 from http://www.nursing.ucla/edu/staff-members-deborah-koniak-griffin/.

Lange, L. L. (1992). Using clinical data to enhance nursing outcomes. In *Annual WIN Assembly, 6: WIN Handout* (pp. 3-7). Boulder, CO: WIN.

Leininger, M. (1968). The research critique: Nature, Function, and Art. In *Communicating Nursing Research, 1.* Boulder, CO: WCHEN. Reprinted in WIN (2007) *The anniversary book: 50 years of advancing nursing in the West* (pp. 93-103). Portland, OR: WIN.

Leininger, M. (1992). Reflections on WCHEN and *The Research Critique.* In *The anniversary book: A history of nursing in the West 1956-1992* (pp. 43-49). Boulder, CO: WIN.

Living Legends. (2016). American Academy of Nursing. Retrieved February 7, 2017 from http://www.aannet.org/about/fellows/living-legends.

McNeil, P. A., & Lindeman, C. A. (in press). A history of the Western Institute of Nursing and its *Communicating Nursing Research* conferences. *Nursing Research.*

Mitchell, E. S. (2017). Contributor. *Our bodies, ourselves.* Retrieved February 18, 2017 from http://www.ourbodiesourselves.org/about/contributors/ellen-sullivan-mitchell/.

Mitsunaga, B. K. (1992). A turning point in *Communicating Nursing Research.* In *The anniversary book: A history of nursing in the West 1956-1992* (pp. 83-87). Boulder, CO: WIN.

Murdaugh, C. (1992). Research information exchange for clinical agency staff. In *The anniversary book: A history of nursing in the West 1956-1992* (pp. 119-122). Boulder, CO: WIN.

Nichols, E. G. (1992). Networks: Spider webs or snowflakes? In *The anniversary book: A history of nursing in the West 1956-1992* (pp. 131-132). Boulder, CO: WIN.

Pepper, G. A. (1992). The 25th and beyond: Research in the service setting. In *The anniversary book: A history of nursing in the West 1956-1992* (pp. 141-145). Boulder, CO: WIN.

Rawlinson, M. E. (1992). Contributions of posters and symposia to research communication. In *The anniversary book: A history of nursing in the West 1956-1992* (pp. 109-114). Boulder, CO: WIN.

Schwab, J. (1964). Structure of the disciplines: Meanings and significances. In G. W. Ford & L. Pugno (Eds.) *The structure of knowledge and the curriculum.* Chicago, IL: Rand McNally.

Sigma Theta Tau International (STTI). (2017). International nurse researcher hall of fame. Retrieved February 19, 2017 from http://www.nursinglibrary.org/vhl/pages/halloffame_current.html.

Suppe, F. (Ed.). (1977). *The structure of scientific theories.* 2nd Ed. Urbana, IL: University of Illinois Press.

Tilden, V. P. (1992). Beyond the 25th: Nursing research in the future. In *The anniversary book: A history of nursing in the West 1956-1992* (pp. 135-139). Boulder, CO: WIN.

Verran, J. A. (2017). Joyce A. Verran. Retrieved February 18, 2017 from http://www.ucdenver.edu/academics/colleges/nursing/faculty-staff/faculty/Pages/J_verann.aspx.

Ward, M. J. (1992). The compilation of nursing research instruments projects. In *The anniversary book: A history of nursing in the West 1956-1992* (pp. 99-103). Boulder, CO: WIN.

Weinert, C. (2011). Clarann Weinert. Retrieved February 18, 2017 from http://www.montana.edu/cweinert/.

Western Council on Higher Education for Nursing (WCHEN). (1958, March 16-17). *Nursing education: Today, tomorrow, the day after that,* San Francisco, CA. Proceedings. WIN Archives: Portland, OR.

Western Council on Higher Education for Nursing (WCHEN). (1960, March 24-25). *Third annual western conference on nursing education: Nurses for tomorrow: Developing action programs,* Salt Lake City, UT. WIN Archives: Portland, OR.

Western Council on Higher Education for Nursing (WCHEN). (1968). Consultants comments. In *On-going research projects in nursing in the Western region* (p. 47). Boulder, CO: WICHE. WIN Archives, Portland, OR.

Western Institute of Nursing (WIN). (1992). *The anniversary book: A history of nursing in the West 1956-1992.* Boulder, CO: WIN.

Western Institute of Nursing (WIN). (2007). *The anniversary book: 50 years of advancing nursing in the West 1957-2007.* Portland, OR: WIN.

Western Institute of Nursing (WIN). (2017). State of the science speakers. In *Celebrating 50 years of Communicating Nursing Research conferences: Save the date.* Portland, OR: WIN.

Woods, N. F. (2017). Nancy Woods. Retrieved February 18, 2017 from https://nursing.uw.edu/person/nancy-woods/.

Young, H. M. (2017). Heather Young. Retrieved February 19, 2017 from http://www.ucdmc.ucdavis.edu/nursing/ourteam/leadership/youngbio.html.

Young, H. M., Bakewell-Sachs, S., & Sarna, L. (in press). Nursing practice, research, and education in the West: The best is yet to come. *Nursing Research.*

60-YEAR TIMELINE OF THE WCHEN/WIN

THE FIRST DECADE: 1955-1965

American Socio-Political Context
The public is focused on the cold war and the conflict between democracy and communism.

Alaska and Hawaii are granted statehood.

A $1.25 minimum wage law is signed.

John Glenn orbits the earth three times in a space capsule.

President John Kennedy is assassinated.

Lyndon Johnson becomes President of the United States.

Race riots across the country continue.

The Vietnam war begins.

American Health Care/Nursing Context
The President's Commission on Education calls for a 50 percent increase in nurses based on projected population growth.

Some progress is made in working conditions for nurses; shift differentials, overtime and pay by cash rather than maintenance compensation are the norm.

The Nurse Training Act is signed into law.

The American Nurses Association approves a position paper, "Education for Entry into Practice."

Federal traineeships for baccalaureate and graduate studies are made available for eligible nursing students.

Events in Nursing in the West
Harold Enarson is first Director of WICHE.

The young Western Interstate Commission for Higher Education (WICHE) (founded in 1951) moves headquarters from Eugene, OR to Boulder, CO.

WICHE appoints Vera Fry to convene the Western Regional Meeting on Advanced Education for Nursing, which recommends a consultant to study nursing issues in the West.

Helen Nahm is hired as WICHE consultant for nursing. She visits 20 of the 33 colleges and universities in the 13 Western states, interviews 300 persons concerned with nursing, and reports findings.

The Berkley Conference is convened to share the Nahm Report and appoints the first "Committee of Seven."

The Committee of Seven recommends what becomes the creation of the Western Council on Higher Education for Nursing (WCHEN).

Faye Abdellah joins WICHE briefly as a consultant for nursing.

Jo Eleanor Elliott is appointed to lead the nursing program at WCHEN to inspire a collaborative, regional approach to issues in the discipline and the steps necessary to improve practice.

WCHEN is officially organized.

The first annual WCHEN council meeting is held.

Elliott collaborates on three conferences to expand and strengthen nursing research in the West at the University of Colorado, University of California Berkley, and the University of Washington.

Robert Kroepsch becomes second Executive Director of WICHE.

WCHEN Projects
"Continuing Education to Improve Mental Health"
"Changing Nurses' Participation in Health Planning"
"Preparation and Utilization of New Nursing Graduates"
A plan for the *Communicating Nursing Research* conference is begun.
Semi-annual or annual WCHEN council meetings continue.

THE SECOND DECADE: 1966-1975

American Socio-Political Context
The Civil Rights Bill is signed into law.
The United States engages in the war in Vietnam.
Martin Luther King and Robert Kennedy are assassinated.
Postsecondary education experiences significant growth.
Richard Nixon is elected President of the United States and later resigns.
Gerald R. Ford becomes President of the United States.
A population explosion brings new problems: overcrowded schools, increased taxes, congestion, and pollution.
The Equal Rights Amendment (ERA) is introduced federally for state ratification.
Minimum wage is $2.10/hr.

American Health Care/Nursing Context
Medicare legislation is passed.
Cost-Age ratio for medications is $41.40/year for people age 65 and over; average cost for medications is $21/year.
Medical research, improves nutrition, improved housing and living conditions begin to dramatically increased longevity.
Successful organ transplants are achieved.
The Lysaught report, "An Abstract for Action" notes (p. 83): "This commission assumes as a first principle that excellence in nursing practice results in measurable benefits; we are dismayed that so little research has been done on actual effects of nursing intervention and care."
Ava Dilworth, research branch, Division of Nursing, concludes there was no doubt about the need for nursing research, but she doubts that the nursing profession really wanted research as there was no demand for it.
Graduate programs in nursing move to emphasize clinical specialization rather than nursing education or administration.

WCHEN Events
Phillip Sirotkin becomes third Executive Director of WICHE.
The annual *Communicating Nursing Research* conference begins.
The *Communicating Nursing Research* conference structure includes formal critique of research presentations.
Marge Batey produces and edits the *Communicating Nursing Research* proceedings.
The *Western Society for Research in Nursing* is established.

WCHEN Projects
"Today and Tomorrow in Western Nursing," a survey of nursing needs and resources
"Regional Program for Nursing Research Development"

"Delphi Survey of Priorities in Clinical Nursing Research"
"Compilation of Nursing Research Instruments:" became known as *The Blue Book*
"Continuing Education Project for Nurses: Idaho, Montana, Wyoming"
"Models for Introducing Cultural Diversity in Nursing"
"The Effectiveness of the Leadership Program in Nursing"
"Developing a Q-Sort Instrument to Delineate Differences Between Graduates of
    Baccalaureate and Associate Degree Programs"
"Curriculum Improvement"
"Continuing Education in Psychiatric Mental Health Nursing"
"Faculty Development to Meet Minority Group Needs"
"Development of Nurse Faculty for Improving and Expanding Continuing Education
    and In-service Education Programs"
"Analysis and Planning for Improved Distribution of Nursing Personnel and Services"
"Training Nurses to Improve Patient Education"
"Feasibility Study: Leadership Preparation for Complex Organizations"

THE THIRD DECADE: 1976-1985

American Socio-Political Context
Jimmy Carter is elected President of the United States.
The United States economy shifts from an industrial base to an information-based
    economy.
The middle class continues to make economic gains.
Attempts are made to link the high technology explosion with high touch.
The Berlin wall collapses.
For the first time, all Western Europe is governed by democracies.
Leadership shifts from the World War II generation to the Vietnam War generation,
    bringing with it a mistrust of government.
Second wave of feminism emerges.
Wage inequality becomes a rallying cry for women.
Ronald Reagan is elected President of the United States.

American Health Care/Nursing Context
Disease-related groups (DRGs) are introduced as a means to manage health care costs.
Increased professional choices for women affect enrollments in schools of nursing.
Sex discrimination becomes an issue within nursing as men enter the profession in
    greater numbers.
Hospitals, concerned with a perceived lack of psychomotor skills among new nursing
    graduates, initiate longer orientation programs and urge schools of nursing to
    develop "internship" programs.
Increased use of technology in clinical settings and increased acuity level of patients
    in hospital settings results in an increased demand for nurses. This becomes
    known as the "quicker and sicker" phenomenon.
Long-term care and living with chronic conditions becomes a focus in nursing education.
Nursing practice models move from functional assignments to team nursing to
    primary nursing.
Community nursing and nursing centers are re-introduced into education and practice
    settings.

WCHEN Events
Jo Eleanor Elliott leaves WCHEN to become the Director of the federal Division of Nursing.
Following brief leadership by Sally Ruybal, Jeanne Kearns is appointed Director of Nursing Programs at WICHE.
The *Communicating Nursing Research* conference structure eliminates the formal critique and moves to discussion format.
Poster sessions are added to the *Communicating Nursing Research* conference.
Pamela Brink begins the *Western Journal of Nursing Research.*
RIFF-RAFF breaks into the annual research conference.
A new Committee of Seven is appointed to explore the status of the WCHEN organization.
WIN Emeriti status is begun.
The New Researcher Award is established, later names for Carol A. Lindeman.

WCHEN Projects
"Continuing Education to Improve Mental Health"
"Changing Nurses' Participation in Health Planning"
"Preparation and Utilization of New Nursing Graduates"

THE FOURTH DECADE: 1986-1995

American Socio-Political Context
George H. W. Bush is elected President of the United States
Free trade and a global market place boom.
Knowledge workers become the power brokers of the economy.
The wage gap between the rich and the poor continues to grow.
Minimum wage is $4.25/hour.
The United States forms a coalition of nations and engages in the first Gulf war.
The country starts the 1990s with a budget surplus.
China moves toward becoming an economic force in the world.
William J. Clinton is elected President of the United States
A religious revival influences national and local elections.
The U.S. Human Genome Project is begun to identify the approximately 20,000 to 25,000 genes in the human DNA; determine sequences of the 3 billion chemical pairs that make up human DNA; improve tools for data analysis; and address ethical, legal and social issues arising from the project.

American Health Care/Nursing Context
The pharmaceutical industry grows and moves to marketing prescription drugs directly to consumers.
A significant percentage of the population living beyond the age of 85 affects nursing education and health care delivery.
The effect of poverty, absence of health care insurance, and growing health care costs significantly increases the percentage of the GNP spent on health care.
The delivery of health care moves to a business model with an emphasis on competition. In addition there is a move from a fee-based approach to a capitated or managed care approach to financing health care.

144

The expansion of the use of computers in processing, recording, and securing information in clinical nursing practice adds another skill requirement for nursing personnel.

Prospective nursing students grow more concerned with economic rather than service-oriented values.

The debate regarding education for entry into practice between baccalaureate and associate degree nursing programs continues and in some states, escalates.

The inability to balance supply and demand for nursing personnel continues, leading to periods of shortage and surplus.

Independent nursing practices grow as a model of care as do the numbers of Nurse Practitioners in joint practices.

Numbers of nurses from minority groups increase substantially.

WIN Events

Committee of Seven recommends that WCHEN separate from WICHE.

The separation of WCHEN from WICHE is approved and the Western Institute of Nursing (WIN) is born.

Membership with voting privileges in WIN is opened to schools of nursing, health care agencies, and individuals in the West.

The first WIN Assembly meeting is held.

The Western Academy of Nurses is established.

The Jo Eleanor Elliott Leadership Award is established.

The Research Information Exchange is added to the annual *Communicating Nursing Research* conference.

The Distinguished Research Lectureship Award is established.

The Anna M. Shannon Mentorship Award is established.

State of the Art and/or Science Papers are introduced to the *Communicating Nursing Research* conference.

WIN Projects

"Information Concerning the Impact of DRGs in the Reimbursement of Hospitals on Clinical Nursing Care in Both Hospitals and Community Settings"

"A Western Project to Improve Training in Geriatric Nursing"

"Hospital Nursing Characteristics and Nursing Needs in the Western Region"

"Nurse Continuing Education Program: Special Needs of Racial/Ethnic Minority Populations Who Abuse Alcohol and Other Drugs"

"Dissemination of Information Related to Strengthening of Nursing Education and Practice and to Set Future Directions"

THE FIFTH DECADE: 1996-2007

American Socio-Political Context

George W. Bush is elected President of the United States.

The country experiences the attacks of 9/11, 2001.

The war on terrorism and homeland security drive decisions including federal spending priorities.

The surplus of federal funds becomes a deficit.

Scientists agree on the reality of global warming.

The price of oil increases and there is a move to develop alternative energy sources.
Human Genome Project is completed in 2003 with analysis continuing for many years.
Minimum wage is $5.15/hour.

American Health Care/Nursing Context

Health care issues focus on rising costs and the growing number of uninsured.
Medicare expenditures exceed anticipated growth raising concerns about its long-term viability.
The Institute of Medicine releases the following: *To Err is Human: Building a Safer Health System* and *Crossing the Quality Chasm.*
Evidence-based practice becomes the standard for health care.
The generation of nursing knowledge becomes a global activity.

WIN Events

Following a call for proposals, Oregon Health & Science University becomes the host organization and WIN offices move from Boulder, Colorado to Portland, Oregon.
Paula McNeil is appointed Executive Director.
WIN is incorporated as a nonprofit organization under Oregon law.
The annual WIN assembly continues and is renamed the WIN Member Assembly.
The *Communicating Nursing Research* conference continues with all-time high increases in attendance.
Poster awards are established at the conference for individual and student members and for participants in the Research & Information Exchange.
Research grants for WIN members are established and jointly funded by WIN, Sigma Theta Tau International, the American Nurses Foundation, and generous donations by WIN members.
WIN collaborates to form the Council for the Advancement of Nursing Science.
Dissertation award is established in conjunction with the Council for the Advancement of Nursing Science.
The Patsy A. Perry Award for Physiological Nursing Research Award is established.
The WIN/John A. Hartford Foundation Regional Geriatric Nursing Research Award is established.

WIN Projects

Website, www.nursingPhD.org, is initiated as a resource for prospective doctoral students.
NEXus - The Nursing Education Xchange: Partnering to increase the capacity of nursing doctoral programs
"Improving Healthcare through Nursing Informatics"
"Leadership Development Initiative" begins, later named the Clinical Inquiry Initiative

---

THE SIXTH DECADE: 2007-2017

American Socio-Political Context

The first African American, Barack Obama, is elected President of the United States; holds office for eight years.
The United States recovers from global economic crisis and recession.
Minimum wage, equal pay, and wage transparency legislation are introduced.
Minimum wage is $7.25/hour.

The country and the world fight radical extremist terrorism.
An anti-government movement strengthens
Social Media emerge as a major means of communication.
Donald J. Trump is elected President of the United States.

American Health Care/Nursing Context
The Affordable Care Act (ACA), "Obamacare," is passed, providing an increase in
number of Americans covered by health insurance.
Though American health care costs slowed under the ACA, they continue to exceed
those compared with other advanced nations of the world while outcomes fall
short.
The Institute of Medicine releases *The Future of Nursing: Leading Change,
Advancing Health*.
Doctor of Nursing Practice (DNP) programs grow throughout the country.
Informatics emerges as a major influence in health care practice.
Health care practice focuses on quality, safety, and outcomes.
Continuation of the ACA is threatened by Republican control of all three branches of
government in 2017.

WIN Events
The Ann M. Voda American Indian/Alaskan Native/First Nation Conference Award is
established.
The WIN/John A. Hartford Foundation Regional Geriatric Nursing Education Award
is established.
The dissertation award is established in collaboration with the Council on the
Advancement of Nursing Science (CANS).

WIN Projects
50X50 Fundraising Project in which over $50,000 was raised by the 50th Anniversary
of the Communicating Nursing Research conference.
The first award of $10,000, jointly sponsored by Sigma Theta Tau International, was
announced at the 50th anniversary of the Communicating Nursing Research
Conference.
Work to establish an endowment fund begins in order to continue increasing the
amount and number of grant awards.
A task force is named to facilitate organizational efforts in development and
membership recruitment/retention.

Appendix A
Communicating Nursing Research **Conference Keynote Addresses**

1968   Madeleine Leininger, University of Washington
The Research Critique: Nature, Function, & Art

1969   Katherine J. Hoffman, University of Washington
Problem Identification & the Research Design

1970   Marjorie V. Batey, University of Washington
Methodological Issues in Research

1971   None

1972   R. Maureen Maxwell, Loma Linda University
The Many Sources of Nursing Knowledge

1973   Jeanne Q. Benoliel, University of Washington
Collaboration & Competition in Nursing

1974   Patricia M. MacElveen, University of Washington
Critical Issues in Access to Data

1975   Dorothy L. McLeod, Arizona State University
Nursing Research Priorities: Choice or Chance

1976   Rheba de Tornyay, University of Washington
Nursing Research in the Bicentennial Year

1977   Sue K. Donaldson & Dorothy M. Crowley, University of Washington
Discipline of Nursing: Structure & Practice

1978   Marjorie V. Batey, University of Washington
Research Communication: Its Functions, Audience, & Media

1979   Susan R. Gortner, University of California, San Francisco
Nursing Science in Transition

1980   Carol A. Lindeman, Oregon Health & Science University
The Challenge of Nursing Research in the 1980s

1981   Betty K. Mitsunaga, University of Colorado Health Science Center
The Use of Knowledge and Health Policy Planning: Forms & Functions of the Relationships

1982   Kathryn E. Barnard, University of Washington
The Research Cycle: Nursing, the Profession, the Discipline

1983   Ada Sue Hinshaw, University of Arizona
The Image of Nursing Research: Issues & Strategies

1984   Jeanne Quint Benoliel, University of Washington
Advancing Nursing Science: Qualitative Approaches

Jan R. Atwood, University of Arizona
Advancing Nursing Science: Quantitative Approaches

1985   Linda K. Amos, University of Utah
Influencing the Future of Nursing Research through Power & Politics

1986   Nancy Fugate Woods, University of Washington
The Winds of Change

1987   Jean Watson, University of Colorado Health Science Center
Academic and Clinical Collaboration: Advancing the Art & Science of Human Caring

Sue T. Hegyvary, University of Washington
Collaboration in Nursing Research: Advancing the Science of Human Care

1988   Anne J. Davis, University of California, San Francisco
Nursing: A Socially Responsible Profession

1989   Carol A. Lindeman, Oregon Health & Science University
Choices within Challenges

1990   Jo Eleanor Elliott, (Former) Division of Nursing, USPHS
Nursing Research: Transcending the 20th Century

1991   Jane S. Norbeck, University of California, San Francisco
The Merging of Agendas for Education, Research, & Practice

WIN Keynote: Doris Kearns Goodwin, Pulitzer Historian & Presidential Biographer
A Look at the Private Lives of Our Public Figures

1992   Carol A. Lindeman, Oregon Health & Science University
The New Scholarship

Plenary: Ada Sue Hinshaw, University of Arizona
The Impact of Nursing Science on Health Policy

WIN Address: Linda L. Lange, University of Utah
Using Clinical Data to Enhance Nursing Outcomes

1993   Sue T. Hegyvary, University of Washington
Scholarship for Practice in a Changing World

WIN Keynote: Sanford Levy, Montana State University
Moral Theory & Moral Practice: A Philosopher's Perspective

WIN Keynote: Anne R. Bavier, Agency for Health Care Policy & Research, USPHS
Research, Practice, & Education within the Health Care Agenda

1995   Janet A. Rodgers, University of San Diego
Innovation & Collaboration: Responses to Health Care Needs–Implications for Nursing

1996   Juanita S. Tate, University of Colorado Health Science Center
Advancing Nursing in Turbulent Times: Implications for Practice, Education, & Research

1997   Sue T. Hegyvary, University of Washington
Nursing: Changing the Environment

1998   Barbara Durand, Arizona State University
Quality Research for Quality Practice

1999   Mary Ann Curry, Oregon Health & Science University
Strategy & Serendipity: Using Research to Influence Health Policy

2000   Colleen J. Goode, University of Colorado Hospital, Denver
Building on a Legacy of Excellence in Nursing Research: Evidence-Based Practice

Barbara Valanis, Kaiser Permanente Center for Health Research. Portland, OR
Thinking Downstream: Research Evidence-Based Practice in Managed Care

2001   Mary A. Blegen, University of Colorado Health Science Center
Health Care Challenges Beyond 2001: Nursing Staffing for Quality of Care

Betty Bierut Gallucci, University of Washington
Genomics, Pharmacogenetics, & Proteomics: New Era Methodologies for Nursing Research

2002   Yvonne Maddox, National Institute of Child Health & Human Development, NIH
Health Disparities: Meeting the Challenge

2003   Geraldine (Polly) Bednash American Association of Colleges of Nursing
Rediscovering Nursing: The Societal Imperative to Evolve & Change

2004   Marie J. Cowan, University of California Los Angeles
Hallmarks of Quality: Generating & Using Knowledge

Marita G. Titler, University of Iowa Hospitals & Clinics
Translation Science: Quality, Methods, & Issues

2005   Melanie C. Dreher, Rush University
Redesigning Nursing Education

2006   Bernadette M. Melnyk, Arizona State University
Transforming Health Care from the Inside Out: Knowledge to Advance Evidence-Based Practice in Clinical & Educational Settings

2007   50th Anniversary of WIN
Education: Christine A. Tanner, Oregon Health & Science University
Respondents:
Carol A. Ashton, Idaho State University
Patricia Benner, University of California, San Francisco

Practice: Marie J. Driever, Providence Portland Medical Center. OR
Respondents:
Julie McNulty, Alaska Native Medical Center, Anchorage
Nancy Nowak, Intermountain Healthcare, Salt Lake City, UT
Lorie R. Wild, University of Washington Medical Center

Research: Margaret Heitkemper, University of Washington
Respondents:
Cindy Mendelson, University of New Mexico
Adeline M. Nyamathi, University of California, Los Angeles

2008   Pamela H. Mitchell, University of Washington
Knowledge That Matters: Integrating Research, Practice, & Education

2009   Mary L. "Nora" Disis, University of Washington School of Medicine
*CTSAs: An Interdisciplinary Approach to Improving Patient Care—
T1 Translation in an Academic Environment: Breast Cancer Vaccine
Development*

2010   Nancy Ridenour, University of New Mexico
Integrating Practice, Research, & Education with Policy

2011   Michael R. Bleich, Oregon Health & Science University
*The Research Imperative and the IOM Future of Nursing: Strengthening
Nursing's Contribution to Leading Change and Advancing Health*

2012   Kathi Mooney, University of Utah
*The Innovative Way: Insights Drawn from Creativity, Flow, & Serendipity to
Advance Nursing Science*

2013   Heather M. Young, University of California, Davis
Nurses Leading Change, Advancing Health: Our Campaign for Action

2014   David Shoultz, The Bill and Melinda Gates Foundation, Seattle, WA
Nursing and Health: A Global Perspective

2015   Barbara J. Safriet, Lewis & Clark Law School, Portland, OR
Equity & Access: Melding Policy with Nursing Research, Practice, & Education

2016   George Demiris, University of Washington
Informatics Tools for Patient Engagement

2017   Doris Kearns Goodwin, Pulitzer Prize Winner and Presidential Historian
Leadership Lessons from the White House

Appendix B
Communicating Nursing Research **Conference Distinguished Research Lectureship**

1988   Ramona T. Mercer, University of California San Francisco
      The Ps & Qs of Mounting & Maintaining a Research Career

1989   Jeanne Q. Benoliel, University of Washington
      From Research to Scholarship: Challenges, Choices, & Transitions

1990   Agnes M. Aamodt, University of Arizona
      *Toward Conceptualizations in Nursing: Harbingers from the Sciences &
      Humanities*

1991   Patricia G. Archbold, Oregon Health & Science University
      An Interdisciplinary Approach to Family Caregiving Research

1992   Plenary Address: Ada Sue Hinshaw, National Center for Nursing Research
      The Impact of Nursing Science on Health Policy

1993   Nancy F. Woods, University of Washington
      Women's Lives, Women's Health

1994   Adeline Nyamathi, University of California Los Angeles
      A Research Trajectory: An Evolving Process

1995   Joyce A. Verran, University of Arizona
      Career Ingredients: Windows and Wagers; Wards and Wizards

1996   Marie J. Cowan, University of Washington
      *Myocardial Infarction and its Impact from the Cellular to the Community
      Level: Nineteen Years of Study*

1997   William L. Holzemer, University of California San Francisco
      The Challenge of Measuring the Quality of Nursing Care

1998   Margaret Heitkemper, University of Washington
      A Biopsychosocial Model of Irritable Bowel Syndrome

1999   Marylin J. Dodd, University of California San Francisco
      Self-Care: Not as Simple as We Hoped

2000   Leona L. Eggert, University of Washington
      *Science Based Prevention Approaches to Promoting Healthy Adolescent
      Behaviors*

      Virginia Tilden, Oregon Health & Science University
      Dying and How I Got There: A Research Journey

2001   Lillian M. Nail, Oregon Health & Science University
      *From Curiosity to Advocacy: Developing a Program of Research on Coping
      with Cancer Treatment*

2002   Kathleen Dracup, University of California San Francisco
Beyond the Patient: Caring for Families

2003   Ida M. (Ki) Moore, University of Arizona
Surviving Childhood Leukemia: Contributions and Challenges of CNS Treatment

2004   Pamela H. Mitchell, University of Washington
Biobehavioral Nursing Research: It's All about Systems

2005   Frances Marcus Lewis, University of Washington
Family-Focused Research in Nursing Science: Why Is It Important to Do This Work?

2006   Christine Miaskowski, University of California San Francisco
The Ten Commandments of Research: The Nurse Scientist's Perspective

2007   Maureen R. Keefe, University of Utah
Coming of Age in the Western Institute of Nursing

2008   Clarann Weinert, Montana State University
One Successful Nursing Research Career: The 5 Ps and More

2009   Elaine Adams Thompson, University of Washington
Intersection of Nursing Science & Prevention Science: Promoting Healthy Adolescent Development

2010   Ginette A. Pepper, University of Utah
Bridges on the River Why

2011   Bernadette M. Melnyk, Arizona State University
The "So What" Factor in a Time of Healthcare Reform: Conducting Research & EbP Projects That Impact Healthcare Quality, Cost, and Patient Outcomes

2012   Martha J. Lentz, University of Washington
Sleep: Now That Is an Interesting Topic

2013   Terry A. Badger, University of Arizona
Psychological Distress, Dyadic Interdependence, and Cancer Survivorship

2014   Deborah Koniak-Griffin, University of California Los Angeles
Maintaining Focus as the Pendulum Swings: A Program of Research with Teen Parents

2015   Judith G. Baggs, Oregon Health & Science University
Collaborative Care and Inter-Professional Education: A 30-Year Research Journey

2016   Carrie J. Merkle, University of Arizona
Inflammation: More Than a Response to Injury

2017   Joan Shaver, University of Arizona
A Journey through Women's Health and Sleep Science: Then, Now and Imagine!

Appendix C
Carol A. Lindeman Award for a New Researcher Award

The WCHEN/WIN Annual Award for Achievement of a New Researcher was established in 1976 and supported through 1987 by Carol A. Lindeman. The award was then renamed the Carol A. Lindeman Award for a New Researcher to recognize Dr. Lindeman's contributions to nursing research and commitment to the organization.

1978   Alice S. Demi, University of Colorado Medical Center
       Adjustment to Widowhood after a Sudden Death: Suicide and Non-suicide Survivors Compared

1979   Joanne Sullivan Marut, University of California San Francisco
       A Comparison of Primiparas' Perceptions of Vaginal & Cesarean Births

1980   Carolyn Webster-Stratton, University of Washington
       Modification of Mothers' Behaviors and Attitudes through Parent Education Based on Videotape Modeling

1981   Susan J. Quaal, Veterans Administration Medical Center, Salt Lake City, Utah
       A Study of Fitness and Cardiovascular Risk Factors in Male Office Workers

1982   Letha Lierman, University of Utah
       Psychological Preparation and Supportive Care for Mastectomy Patients

1983   Diane Magyary, University of Washington
       Cross-Time and Cross-Situational Comparisons of Mother-Preterm Infant Interactions

1984   Shawn K. Elmore, University of Washington
       The Moderating Effect of Social Support upon Depression

1985   Pam Hellings, Oregon Health & Science University
       A Discriminant Model to Predict Breast Feeding Success

1986   Gwenyth G. Gerhard, University of Lowell, MA
       Predicting Acute Surgical Pain from Habitual Physical Activity

1987   Frederica W. O'Connor, University of Washington
       Increasing Surgical Teaching

1988   Kären M. Landenburger, University of Colorado
       Conflicting Realities of Women in Abusive Relationships

1989   Sally H. Rankin, University of California San Francisco
       Women as Patients & Women as Caregivers: Difficulties in Recovery from Cardiac Surgery

1990   JoAnn G. Congdon, University of Colorado Health Sciences Center
       Managing the Incongruities: An Analysis of Hospital Discharge of the Elderly

1991   Diana J. Wilkie, University of Washington
        Lung Cancer Pain Coping Strategies

1992   Jane M. Georges, University of Washington
        Distressing Gastrointestinal Symptoms in Postmenopausal Women

1993   Patricia E. Stevens, University of California San Francisco
        Health Care Interactions as Experienced by Clients: Lesbian's Narratives

1994   Debra Gay Anderson, Washington State University Vancouver
        Homeless Women: The Perceptions of Families of Origin

1995   Patricia A. Carney, Dartmouth Medical School, Hanover, NH
        *HIV Prevention: Do Nurse Practitioners and Physicians Provide Equivalent
        Care?*

1996   JoAnn Perry, University of British Columbia, Vancouver, BC, Canada
        Family Know-How as Interpretive Caring: Caregiving in Alzheimer's Disease

1997   Elizabeth A. LeCuyer, Washington State University Vancouver
        Maternal Sensitivity and Responsiveness in the Transition to Toddlerhood

1998   Gretchen M. Zunkel, Arizona State University
        Relational Coping Following Early Stage Breast Cancer Diagnosis

1999   Irene S. Morgan, California State University Chico
        *Health Promotion in Midlife Women: A Grounded Theory of Influencing
        Processes*

2000   Christine A. Thurston, Oregon Health Plan, Department of Human Services,
        Salem, OR
        Recovering Women: A Narrative Inquiry of Self & Belonging in Women

2001   Lori A. Loan, Madigan Army Medical Center, Tacoma, WA
        Ventilator Inspired Gas Temperature and Tracheal Injury in Neonates

2002   Mary Jayne Johnson, Brigham Young University, Provo, UT
        *The Medication-Taking Questionnaire for Measuring Patterned Behavior
        Adherence*

2003   Kuei-Hsiang Hsueh, Northern Arizona University, Flagstaff, AZ
        Family Caregiving Experience among Chinese Caregivers in the United States

2004   Kristin F. Lutz, Oregon Health & Science University
        Living Two Lives: A Grounded Theory of Abuse during Pregnancy

        Young-Shin Lee, University of San Diego
        Motivation and Physical Activity among Older Adults

2005   Patricia Flannery Pearce, University of Utah
        Designing with Children, for Children: Computerized Activity Recall

156

2006   Margaret F. Clayton, University of Utah
       Communication with Breast Cancer Survivors

2007   Catherine R. Van Son, Oregon Health & Science University
       Ethnomedicine Use by Older Adults from a Slavic Community

2008   Cecelia I. Roscigno, University of Washington
       Longing for Everydayness: Life after Traumatic Brain Injury in Children

2009   Gwen Latendresse, University of Utah
       Maternal Use of Mood Disorder Medication Predicts the Occurrence of Preterm Birth

2010   Katie Anne Adamson, Washington State University, Spokane, WA
       Comparing Learning Outcomes between Two Experiential Teaching Strategies

2011   Connie Kim Yen Nguyen-Truong, Oregon Health & Science University
       Translation Team Approach: Psychometrics of a Vietnamese PAP Testing Survey

2012   Terri L. Yost, Tripler Army Med Center, Honolulu, HI
       Qigong as a Novel Intervention for Service Members with Mild Traumatic Brain Injury

2013   Gayle J. Kipnis, California State University Chico
       Effects of Altitude and Sleep on Perinatal Outcomes

2014   Carolyn Montoya, University of New Mexico
       Children's Self-Perceptions of Weight in a Rural Hispanic Community

2015   Moonju Lee, University of Arizona
       Colorectal Cancer Screening Behaviors among Korean Americans

2016   Lindsey M. Miller, Oregon Health & Science University
       Decision-Making Involvement of Hospitalized Patients with Dementia: A Dyadic Study

2017   Manu Thakral, Kaiser Permanente Washington Health Research Institute, Seattle, WA
       Impact of Opioid Safety Initiatives in Those at High Risk for Opioid-Related Problems

Appendix D
Communicating Nursing Research Conference State-of-Science &
Other Special Addresses

1968 **Introduction:**
Kevin P. Bunnell, WICHE Associate Director
Introduction:
Katherine Hoffman, University of Washington
Follow-up:
Imogene King, Assistant Chief, Research Grants Branch, Division of Nursing
Conclusion:
Maureen Maxwell, Loma Linda University

1969 **Introduction:**
Development of Communicating Nursing Research Series
R. Maureen Maxwell, Loma Linda University
Response to the Conference:
Anne J. Davis, University of California San Francisco
Looking Ahead:
R. Maureen Maxwell, Loma Linda University

1970 **Introduction:**
R. Maureen Maxwell, Loma Linda University
Commentary on Research Facilitation:
Kathryn M. Smith, Chair, WCHEN
Summary of Conference:
R. Maureen Maxwell, Loma Linda University

1971 **Conclusion:**
Marjorie V. Batey, University of Washington

1972 **The Many Faces of Nursing Research:**
Dorothy McLeod, Arizona State University

1973 **Reflections: And the Way Ahead:**
Marjorie V. Batey, University of Washington

1974 **Variety of Sources of Nursing Research Data** (Posthumously published):
Dorothy M. Martin, Loma Linda University

1975 – 1977 None

1978 **Summary Paper:**
The Paradoxical Nature of Nursing Research
Ruth S. Ludemann, Montana State University

1979 **Summarizing Remarks:**
Ada Jacox, University of Colorado

1980 **Closing Remarks:**
Directions for the 1980s: Concerns and Pragmatic Implications
Jean L. J. Lum, University of Hawaii

1981 **Closing Remarks:**
Health Policy and Research Revisited
Anna M. Shannon, Montana State University

1982 – 1989 None

1990 **Closing Address:**
Toward the 21st Century: Nursing Theory, Research, and Practice
Peggy L. Chinn, University of Utah

Special Focus Session: Substance Abuse
Marylou McAthie, Sonoma State University, California
Mary Haack, Guest Researcher, National Institutes of Health
Donna B. Jensen, Oregon Health & Science University
Juanita F. Murphy, Arizona State University
Constance C. Connell, Arizona Board of Nursing
Elizabeth M. Pace, N.U.R.S.E.S. of Colorado Corporation

1991 None

1992 **Podium "State of the Art Papers":**
If Not Now, Then When? Nursing's Research Utilization Imperative
Nancy E. Donaldson, University of California Irvine Medical Center

Measurement: A Foundation of Nursing Science
William L. Holzemer, University of California San Francisco

Nursing Research Serving the Underserved: Homeless Health Care
Ada M. Lindsey, University of California Los Angeles

Attending to Many Voices: Beyond the Qualitative-Quantitative Dialectic
Phyllis R. Schultz, University of Washington

Round Table Discussion Leaders on State of Art Papers:
Ethics Research
Kathleen Chafey, Montana State University
Children's Health
Nancy Hester, University of Colorado Health Science Center
Health Promotion Research
Shirley Cloutier Laffrey, University of Texas, Austin
Organizational and Administration Research
Ruth S. Ludemann, Arizona State University
Cultural Diversity Research
Afaf I. Meleis, University of California San Francisco
Mental Health Research

Helen Nakagawa-Kogan, University of Washington
Physiological Research
Patsy A. Perry, Arizona State University
Gerontological Research
Linda R. Phillips, University of Arizona
Women's Health Research
Nancy F. Woods, University of Washington

1993 **State of the Art & Science Papers:**
State of the Art in Quality of Life Research
Cardiovascular Disease in Women: State of the Science
Geraldine V. Padilla, University of California Los Angeles
Carolyn Murdaugh, National Center of Nursing Research

1994 **WSRN State of the Science Papers:**
Nursing Informatics: State of the Science
Suzanne Bakken Henry, University of California San Francisco
Rural Nursing: Legacy, Science, Trajectory
Clarann Weinert, Montana State University

1995 **WSRN State of the Science Papers:**
Outcomes Research: Examining Clinical Effectiveness
Patricia Moritz, National Institute of Nursing Research
Research in Nursing Distance Education: Defining the Elephant
Dianna Shomaker, University of New Mexico

1996 **WSRN State of the Science Papers:**
Predictive Modeling: Have We Hit the Bull's-Eye or Are the Arrows Flying Free?
Sandra L. Ferketich, University of Arizona
Psychosocial Approaches in Prevention Science: Facing the Challenge with High Risk Youth
Leona L. Eggert, University of Washington

1997 **State of the Science Papers:**
Capturing Nursing's Contribution to Patient Care: An Informatics Approach
Suzanne Bakken Henry, University of California San Francisco
Skeletal Muscle Atrophy and Fatigue
Christine E. Kasper, University of California Los Angeles

Report from 1996 Glaxo Wellcome Inc. Research Award Recipient:
Changing Elderly Patients' Behavior Regarding Medication Management
Rebecca W. Dahl, Carondelet Health Network, Tucson, AZ

1998 **State of the Science Papers:**
Clinical Judgment and Evidence-Based Practice: Conclusions and Controversies
Christine A. Tanner, Oregon Health & Science University
Dying in America: Ethics and End-of-Life Care
Virginia P. Tilden, Oregon Health & Science University
Evaluating Outcomes in a Managed Care Environment
Gerri Lamb, Carondolet Health Care, Tucson, AZ

1999 **State of the Science:**
Current Perspectives in Psychoneuroimmunology for Nursing Research
Carol A. Landis, University of Washington

2000 **State of the Science Symposia:**
Advancing Women's Health Care across the Lifespan
Overview: Advancing Women's Health Care across the Lifespan
Margaret M. Heitkemper, University of Washington
Advancing Knowledge of Biobehavioral Phenomenon for Women's Health
Martha J. Lentz, University of Washington
Carol A. Landis, University of Washington
Advancing Knowledge of Sociocultural Environments for Women's Health
Marcia Killien, University of Washington
Barbara McGrath, University of Washington

The Ever Evolving Science of Symptom Management
Through the Looking Glass: Using Evidence to Frame Practice
Susan Janson, University of California San Francisco
Sleepy or Weepy: The Postpartum Symptom Experience
Kathryn A. Lee, University of California San Francisco
Symptom Clusters and Their Effects on Patients' Outcomes
Marylin Dodd, University of California San Francisco
Christine Miaskowski, University of California San Francisco
Steven M. Paul, University of California San Francisco

2001 **State of the Science Symposium:**
Research Training: Nursing Care for Older People and Populations
Patricia G. Archbold, Oregon Health & Science University
Barbara J. Stewart, Oregon Health & Science University
Beverly Hoeffer, Oregon Health & Science University
Community-Based Intervention Research: Lessons Learned and Thoughts on the State of the Science
Linda R. Phillips, University of Arizona

2002 **State of the Science Papers:**
Health Disparities Research: From Concept to Practice
Jacquelyn H. Flaskerud, University of California Los Angeles
Lessons from the Past, Solutions for the Future: The Millennium Nursing Shortage
Anne M. McNamara, Arizona Hospital & Healthcare Association
Rural Nursing Research: Riddle, Rhyme, Reality
Clarann Weinert, Montana State University

2003 **State of the Science Papers:**
Evidence Base for the Societal Imperative of Patient Safety
Ginette A. Pepper, University of Utah
Progress in the Measurement of Pain as a Multi-Dimensional Subjective Phenomenon
Diana J. Wilkie, University of Illinois

2004 **State of the Science Papers:**
Hallmarks of Quality: Generating Knowledge to Assist Consumers of Long-Term Care
JoAnn G. Congdon, University of Colorado Health Sciences Center
Psychoeducational Interventions for Cancer Pain Serve as a Model for Behavioral Research
Christine Miaskowski, University of California San Francisco

2005 **State of the Science Papers:**
The Science Related to the Work Environment in Acute Care Hospitals
Colleen J. Goode, University of Colorado Hospital
Complementary-Alternative Therapies: From Pseudo to Serious Science
Marlaine C. Smith, University of Colorado at Denver & Health Sciences Center
Innovations in Neonatal Research: You've Come a Long Way Baby
Karen A. Thomas, University of Washington

2006 **State of the Science Papers:**
Early Childhood Obesity in Latino Families: Assembling Knowledge for Practice
Lauren Clark, University of Colorado at Denver Health Sciences Center
State of the Heart: Building Science to Improve Women's Cardiovascular Health
Anne Rosenfeld, Oregon Health & Science University

2007 none (anniversary year)

2008 **State of the Science:**
Health Care Transitions of Youth with Special Health Care Needs: The Never Ending Journey
Cecily L. Betz, University of Southern California
Advances in Nursing Education: Virtual Experiential Communities
Jean Foret Giddens, University of New Mexico
Thoughts about the State of the Science Related to Culturally Competent Care for Persons with Chronic Illness and its Relationships to Practice
Linda R. Phillips, University of California Los Angeles

2009 **State of the Science:**
Practice-Based Evidence vs. Evidence-Based Practice: What is in Our Future?
Susan D. Horn, Institute for Clinical Outcomes Research, Salt Lake City, UT
Partnering with Consumers to Design Health Promotion Research
Deborah Koniak-Griffin, University of California Los Angeles
Opportunities and Challenges in Symptom Clusters Research
Christine Miaskowski, University of California San Francisco
Paula Meek, University of Colorado Denver

2010 **State of the Science:**
Research, Program Evaluation, or QI? Mapping the Edges in Adherence Studies
Paul F. Cook, University of Colorado, Denver, Aurora, CO
Towards Establishing a Qualitative Evidence
Janice M. Morse, University of Utah
Digital Health Consumers: Transforming the Clinical Research Landscape
Huong G. Nguyen, University of Washington

2011 **State of the Science Papers:**
Quality and Safety Competencies in Nursing Education: State of the Science
Amy J. Barton, University of Colorado, Aurora
An Integrative Review of Research on Nursing Handoffs in Acute Care Settings
Nancy Staggers, University of Maryland
Research Methods for Complexity: From the Traditional to the Unique
Joyce A. Verran, University of Colorado, Aurora

2012 **State of the Science Papers:**
Randomized Trials for Comparative Effectiveness: The Bronze Standard Again?
Gary Donaldson, University of Utah
Social Media and Health Care: Where's the Evidence? The Social Media Landscape in Health Care
Diane J. Skiba, University of Colorado, Aurora
Advancing the National Research Priorities in Improvement
Kathleen R. Stevens, University of Texas Health Science Center at San Antonio

2013 **State of the Science Papers:**
Future of Nursing Education: Trends and Innovations
Maureen R. Keefe, University of Utah
Biobehavioral Nursing Science: Landscapes and Horizons—Where Mind Meets Body
Joan L. F. Shaver, University of Arizona
Creating Nursing's Future: Translating Research into Evidence-Based Policy
Marla J. Weston, American Nurses Association
Kathleen M. White, Johns Hopkins University
Cheryl A. Peterson, American Nurses Association

2014 **State of the Science Papers:**
Bridging the Gap: Strengthening Nursing Practice in Low-Resource Countries
R. Kevin Mallinson, George Mason University
Going Global: Past Decade of Nurse-Led Intervention Research in Developing Countries
Adeline M. Nyamathi, University of California Los Angeles
Innovations in Nursing in Resource-Constrained Settings
Joachim G. Voss, University of Washington

2015 **State of the Science Papers:**
Improving Access and Equity in Undergraduate Nursing Education through Academic Partnerships: A Generation of Implementation
Paula Gubrud, Oregon Health & Science University
Dimensions of Access as It Pertains to Best Practices and Health Equity
Sandra L. Haldane, Alaska Native Tribal Health Consort-Southcentral Foundation, Anchorage
Urban as a Determinant of Health: Implications for Nursing Practice and Research
David Vlahov, University of California San Francisco

2016 **State of the Science Papers:**
Innovative Technologies to Promote Patient Engagement Research
Bonnie Gance-Cleveland, University of Colorado, Anschutz Medical Campus
Getting Engaged: A New Paradigm of Research Done Differently
Debra J. Barksdale, Virginia Commonwealth University, Richmond
Evidence Based Design for Behavioral Interventions
Kate Lorig, Stanford University, Palo Alto, California

2017 **State of the Science Papers:**
The Future of Nursing Research in the West: The Best is Yet to Come
Linda Sarna, University of California Los Angeles
The Next 50 Years of Nursing Leadership in the Western States: Visionary Education as Multiplier for WIN.
Heather Young, University of California Davis, Sacramento, CA
Nursing Practice and Advancing Healthcare Transformation
Susan Bakewell-Sachs, Oregon Health & Science University

Appendix E
Western Academy of Nurses
In the *Communicating Nursing Research* **Conference**

In 1989, the Western Academy of Nurses was established to recognize and honor nurses who have demonstrated excellence in nursing practice and have advanced practice in direct care, education, or research. Candidates must be nominated by two WIN members, be a member in good standing of WIN, have been actively engaged in WIN over a period of at least five years, and have demonstrated excellence in scholarship/research, practice, and/or education.

1990: Charter Members
Marci Catanzaro, University of Washington, Seattle, WA
Anna Shannon, Montana State University, Bozeman, MT
Clarann Weinert, Montana State University, Bozeman, MT

1991
Jan Martin, University of Northern Colorado, Greeley, CO
Maryann Pranulis, University of California Los Angeles, Los Angeles, CA
Barbara Trehearne, Group Health Cooperative of Puget Sound, Seattle, WA

1992
Chiyoko Furukawa, University of New Mexico, Albuquerque, NM
Lois Van Cleve, Loma Linda University, Loma Linda, CA

1993
Janelle C. Krueger, Arizona State University, Tempe, AZ

1994
Pamela Baj, San Francisco State University, San Francisco, CA
Marie Driever, Providence Medical Center, Portland, OR
Mary Ann Johnson, Salt Lake City VA Center, University of Utah, Salt Lake City, UT
Heather M. Young, Ida Culver House and University of Washington, Seattle, WA

1995
Janet Bostrom, Stanford Medical Center, Palo Alto, CA
Ruth S. Ludemann, Arizona State University, Tempe, AZ
Pat A. Perry, Arizona State University, Tempe, AZ
Helen B. Ripple, University of California San Francisco Medical Center, San Francisco, CA
Elaine Sorensen Marshall, Brigham Young University, Provo, UT

1996
Carol Ashton, Salt Lake Valley Hospitals, Salt Lake City, UT
Dianne Helmer, Lucile Slater Packard Children's Hospital at Stanford, CA
Julie Johnson, University of Nevada-Reno, Reno, NV
Jeanne Kearns, Former WIN Executive Director, Boulder, CO
Dianna Shomaker, University of New Mexico, Albuquerque, NM

1997
Carol A. Lindeman, Oregon Health & Science University, Portland, OR

1998
Marie Scott Brown, Oregon Health & Science University, Portland, OR
Sandra Ferketich, University of New Mexico, Albuquerque, NM
Ellen M. Lewis, University of California Irvine, Irvine, CA
Diane Peters, University of Northern Colorado, Greeley, CO

1999
Lea Acord, Montana State University, Bozeman, MT
Lynn Clark Callister, Brigham Young University, Provo, UT
Yeou-Lan Duh Chen, Westminster College of Salt Lake City, UT
Tina DeLapp, University of Alaska, Anchorage, Anchorage, AK
Beverly Hoeffer, Oregon Health Sciences University, Portland, OR

2000
Terry Badger, The University of Arizona, Tucson, AZ
Carrie Jo Braden, The University of Arizona, Tucson, AZ
Miyong Kim, The Johns Hopkins University, Baltimore, MD
Barbara L. Mandleco, Brigham Young University, Provo, UT
Ellen Sullivan Mitchell, University of Washington, Seattle, WA
Christine A. Tanner, Oregon Health & Science University, Portland, OR
Nancy White, University of Northern Colorado, Greeley, CO

2001
Kathleen Chafey, Montana State University, Bozeman, MT
Alice Running, University of Nevada, Reno, Reno, NV

2003
Joyce A. Verran, The University of Arizona, Tucson, AZ

2004
Margaret Heitkemper, University of Washington, Seattle, WA
Joan (Kathy) Magilvy, University of Colorado Denver, Aurora, CO
Susan Mattson, Arizona State University, Phoenix, AZ
Ginette Pepper, University of Utah, Salt Lake City, UT

2005
Gerri S. Lamb, The University of Arizona, Tucson, AZ
Donna K. McNeese-Smith, University of California Los Angeles, Los Angeles, CA
Christine M. Mumma, University of Alaska, Anchorage, Anchorage, AK
Adeline M. Nyamathi, University of California Los Angeles, Los Angeles, CA
Nancy Fugate Woods, University of Washington, Seattle, WA

2006
Marcia Killien, University of Washington, Seattle, WA
Martha J. Lentz, University of Washington, Seattle, WA
Nancy Lowe, Oregon Health & Science University, Portland, OR

2007
Amy J. Barton, University of Colorado Denver, Aurora, CO
Marie L. Lobo, University of New Mexico, Albuquerque, NM
Anne Marie Kotzer, The Children's Hospital, Denver, CO
Pamela H. Mitchell, University of Washington, Seattle, WA
Anne Rosenfeld, Oregon Health & Science University, Portland, OR

2008
Ann O. Hubbert, University of Nevada, Reno, Reno, NV
Faye Hummel, University of Northern Colorado, Greeley, CO
Maureen Keefe, University of Utah, Salt Lake City, UT
Ann M. Voda, University of Utah, Salt Lake City, UT

2009
Judith Baggs, Oregon Health & Science University, Portland, OR
Deborah Koniak-Griffin, University of California Los Angeles, Los Angeles, CA
Paula Meek, University of Colorado Denver, Aurora, CO

2010
Kathleen Dracup, University of California San Francisco, San Francisco, CA
Shannon Ruff Dirksen, Arizona State University, Phoenix, AZ
Jo Eleanor Elliott, Western Council on Higher Education in Nursing (WCHEN), Boulder, CO
Elizabeth G. Nichols, Montana State University, Bozeman, MT
Patricia Moritz, University of Colorado Denver, Aurora, CO
Susan Shapiro, Emory Healthcare & Emory University, Atlanta, GA

2011
Barbara St. Pierre Schneider, University of Nevada Las Vegas, Las Vegas, NV

2012
Judith A. Berg, The University of Arizona, Tucson, AZ
Lauren Clark, University of Utah, Salt Lake City, UT
Monica E. Jarrett, University of Washington, Seattle, WA
Joan L. Shaver, The University of Arizona, Tucson, AZ
Carolyn Yucha, University of Nevada Las Vegas, Las Vegas, NV

2013
Patricia Graw Butterfield, Washington State University, Spokane, WA
Janice D. Crist, The University of Arizona, Tucson, AZ
Virginia Tilden, University of Nebraska, Omaha, NE; and Oregon Health & Science University, Portland, OR
Joie Whitney, University of Washington, Seattle, WA

2014
Gail M. Houck, University of Washington, Seattle, WA
Marylyn Morris McEwen, The University of Arizona, Tucson, AZ
Ellen Olshansky, University of California Irvine, Irvine, CA
Alyce A. Schultz, Bozeman, MT
Kate Sheppard, The University of Arizona, Tucson, AZ
Donna Velasquez, Arizona State University, Phoenix, AZ

2015
Bronwynne C. Evans, Arizona State University, Phoenix, AZ
Jane H. Lassetter, Brigham Young University, Provo, UT
Carolyn (Carrie) J. Merkle, The University of Arizona, Tucson, AZ

2016
Jane Carrington, The University of Arizona, Tucson, AZ
Cynthia Corbett, Washington State University, Vancouver, WA
Martha Driessnack, Oregon Health & Science University, Portland, OR
Lissi Hansen, Oregon Health & Science University, Portland, OR

2017
Marjorie V. Batey, PhD, RN, FAAN, University of Washington, Seattle, WA
Basia Belza, University of Washington, Seattle, WA
Neva L. Crogan, Gonzaga University, Spokane, WA
Mary de Leon Siantz, University of California, Davis, Sacramento, CA
Linda Lou Sarna, University of California, Los Angeles, CA
Charlene A. Winters, Montana State University, Missoula, MT

Western Academy of Nurses Panels and Presentations
In the *Communicating Nursing Research* Conference

1994
Panel: Commitment for Advancing Nursing
Clarann Weinert, Montana State University
Relationship Between WAN and the WIN Mission and Goals and Paradigms of Change
Marci Catanzaro, Primary Health Care Associates, Seattle, WA
Integrating Scholarship into Advanced Practice
Barbara Trehearne, Group Health Cooperative of Puget Sound, Seattle, WA
Integrating Scholarship into Administration
Chiyoko Furukawa, University of New Mexico
Janelle Krueger, Arizona State University
Facilitating Faculty Research/Scholarship in a Low Resource Environment

1995
Panel: Collaboration: Innovations for Consumers—Education, Practice, and Research
Moderator: Lois Van Cleve, Loma Linda University
Heather M. Young, University of Washington
Collaboration with Consumers
Marie J. Driever, Providence Portland Medical Center, Portland, OR
Focus on Interdisciplinary Teamwork: A New Form of Collaboration?
Mary Ann Johnson, Salt Lake Veterans Affairs/University of Utah
Collaboration within Education
Pamela A. Baj, San Francisco State University
Effective Models of Research Collaboration

1996
Panel: Adventures in New Ventures
Janet Bostrom, President, Quick Study, Inc.
Developing a Cost Effective Software Solution to the Problem of Regulatory Staff Training

Dianne C. Helmer, Lucile Salter Packard Children's Hospital at Stanford, Palo Alto, CA
Creating a Health Promotion Program to Improve Employee Health in Industry
Dianna Shomaker, University of New Mexico
Developing Distance Education Sites: The Role of the Entrepreneur as Culture Broker
Mary Ann Johnson, Salt Lake Veterans Affairs/University of Utah
Gerontological Nursing: Current and Future Directions

1997
Panel: Nursing 2000 Plus – Through the Wormhole: A Symposium Focusing on Transit Through the Millennium Chaos
Maryann F. Pranulis, University of California San Francisco, CA
Making Sense Out of Nonsense: A Conceptual Framework for Forecasting in an Era of Health Care Paradigm Shift
Carol A. Ashton, Intermountain Healthcare, Urban Central Region Hospitals, Salt Lake City, UT
Being Free to Explore: Flying through the Wormhole to an Enlightened Place
Dianna Shomaker, University of New Mexico
I'm Keen on Interdisciplinary Health Care as Long as I Can Be in Charge!
Marie J. Driever, Providence Portland Medical Center, Portland, OR
Nursing's Contributions to Patient and Health System Needs

1998
Debate: Every Nurse Should be a Nurse Practitioner
Moderator: Dianna Shomaker, University of New Mexico
Pro Argument: Marci Catanzaro, Primary Health Care Associates, Seattle, WA
Con Argument: Mary Ann Johnson, Salt Lake City, VAMC/GRECC, Utah

1999
Panel: Evidence-Based Practice – or "Cookbook" Nursing
Christine A. Tanner, Oregon Health Sciences University, OR
Marie Driever, Providence Portland Medical Center, OR
Patricia Moritz, University of Colorado Health Science Center, Denver, CO
Sheila Quilter Wheeler, President, TeleTriage Systems, San Anselmo, CA

2000
Program: Evidence-Based Practice Y2K: The Strategic Imperative
Nancy Donaldson, University of California San Francisco, CA
Diane Brown, Kaiser Permanente East Bay, Walnut Creek, CA
Lowell Wise, Stanford Hospital & Clinics, Palo Alto, CA

2001
Presentation: Partnerships: Transcending the Boundaries of Knowledge Development and Application
Carol Ashton
President, Health Web Connexions, Salt Lake City, UT
Marie J. Driever
Providence Portland Medical Center, OR
Colleen Keenan
University of California Los Angeles

2002
Presentation: Nursing Clinics: Reducing the Health Disparities of Vulnerable Populations
Terry Badger, University of Arizona
Aaron Strehlow, UCLA SON Health Center at the Union Rescue Mission, Los Angeles, CA
Betty Gale, Arizona State University
Sharon K. Howard, Montana State University

2003
Panel: Best Evidence to Best Practice: How to Get Ready for "Prime Time": Delivery by Design
Marna K. Flaherty-Robb, Oregon Health & Sciences University
Ginette A. Pepper, University of Utah
Diana J. Wilkie, University of Illinois

2006
Program: From Numbers to Knowledge: Leveraging the Power of Nursing Outcome Databases
Nancy Donaldson, University of California San Francisco
Linda Burnes Bolton, Cedar Sinai Medical Center, Los Angeles, CA
Lori A. Loan, Madigan Army Medical Center, Tacoma, WA

2007
Panel: Challenge Papers
Education: Today's Challenge, Tomorrow's Excellence: The Practice of Evidence-Based Education
Roberta J. Emerson, Washington State University, and Kathie Records, Arizona State University
Practice: Sustainability Principles in Nursing
Joachim Voss, University of Washington
Research: Lost in Translation?
Martha Driessnack, University of Iowa

2008
Program: Translating Research Findings into Everyday Clinical Practice
Marilyn P. Chow, Kaiser Permanente, Oakland, CA

2009
Program: Education and Practice: Networks in Innovation
Terry A. Badger, University of Arizona
Patricia D. Horoho, Madigan Army Medical Center, Tacoma, WA
Susan Beck, University of Utah
Joanne Rains Warner, University of Portland, OR

2010
Panel: Impact and Outcomes of Magnet Designation: Patients, Nurses, and Academic Partnerships
Adeline M. Nyamathi, University of California Los Angeles

Anna Gawlinski, University of California Los Angeles Medical Center and School of Nursing
Colleen Goode, University of Colorado Denver, Aurora, CO
Ann Voda, University of Utah

2011
Panel: Strengthening Nursing's Contribution to Leading Change and Improving Health: Perspectives from the California Regional Action Coalition (CA-RAC)
Carol A. Ashton, Idaho State University
Heather M. Young, University of California Davis
Casey R. Shillam, University of California Davis
Nancy E. Donaldson, University of California San Francisco

2012
Panel: Community-Based Participatory Research as a Strategy for Decreasing Health Inequities and Promoting Social Justice
Deborah Koniak-Griffin, University of California Los Angeles
Janna Lesser, University of Texas Health Science Center, San Antonio
Kynna Wright-Volel, University of California Los Angeles
Usha Menon, Arizona State University

2013
Panel: Emerging Gender Science in Cardiovascular Disease
Lynn V. Doering, University of California Los Angeles
Holli A. DeVon, University of Illinois at Chicago
JoAnn Eastwood, University of California Los Angeles
Christopher Sean Lee, Oregon Health & Science University

2014
Panel: Research Innovations in Global Health Nursing
Joie Whitney, University of Washington
Sarah Gimbel, University of Washington
Mary Anne Mercer, Timor-Leste, Health Alliance International, Seattle, WA
Pam Kohler, University of Washington
Julia Robinson, Health Alliance International, Seattle, WA

2015
Panel: Emerging Opportunities for Big Data in Nursing
Moderator: Marylyn McEwen, University of Arizona
John M. Welton, University of Colorado Denver
Blaine Reeder, University of Colorado Denver

2016
Panel: Changing Landscape in the World of Publishing: What Authors Need to Know
Moderator: Deborah Koniak-Griffin, University of California Los Angeles
Steve Clancy, Research Librarian, University of California Irvine
Nancy K. Lowe, Editor-in-Chief, JOGNN, University of Colorado, Anschutz Medical Campus
Jan Morse, Editor, Qualitative Health Research, University of Utah

2017
Panel: Leadership in Omics Education, Practice and Research
Overview: Ginette A. Perry, University of Utah, University of Colorado Denver, Aurora, CO
Education: Charles A. Downs, University of Arizona
Practice: Laura D. Rosenthal, University of Colorado Denver, Aurora, CO
Research: Margaret Heitkemper, University of Washington

Appendix F
Clinical Agencies Participating in the Research and Information Exchange (R&IE) at Communicating Nursing Research

1988
Cedars-Sinai Medical Center, Los Angeles, CA
The Children's Hospital, Denver, CO
Tucson Medical Center, Tucson, AZ
University of California Davis Medical Center, CA
University of California Irvine Medical Center, CA
University Hospital, University of Utah, Salt Lake City, UT
Veterans Administration, Prescott, Arizona

1989
The Children's Hospital, Denver, CO
LDS Hospital, Salt Lake City, UT
University of California Davis Medical Center, CA
University of California Irvine Medical Center, CA
University Hospital, University of Utah, Salt Lake City, UT
Veterans Administration Medical Center, Denver, CO

1990
Boulder Community Hospital, CO
The Children's Hospital, Denver, CO
Group Health Cooperative Central Hospital, Seattle, WA
LDS Hospital, Salt Lake City, UT
Swedish Medical Center, Englewood, CO
University of California Davis Medical Center, CA
University of California Irvine Medical Center, CA
University of California San Diego Medical Center, CA
University Hospital, University of Colorado, CO
University Hospital, University of Utah, Salt Lake City, UT
Veterans Affairs Medical Center, Denver, CO

1991
Carondelet St. Mary's Hospital and Health Center, Tucson, AZ
The Children's Hospital, Denver, CO
LDS Hospital, Salt Lake City, UT
Swedish Medical Center, Englewood, CO
University of California Irvine Medical Center, CA
University of California San Diego Medical Center, CA
University Hospital, University of Colorado, CO
University Hospital, University of Utah, Salt Lake City, UT

1992
Cedars-Sinai Medical Center, Los Angeles, CA
The Children's Hospital, Denver, CO
University of California Irvine Medical Center, CA
Presbyterian/St. Luke's Medical Center, Denver, CO
The Queen's Medical Center, Honolulu, HI

Salt Lake Valley Hospitals: Alta View, Cottonwood, LDS, UT
Sharp Memorial Hospital, San Diego, CA
Stanford University Hospital, CA
Swedish Medical Center, Englewood, CO
University Hospital, Denver, CO

1993
LDS Hospital, Salt Lake City, UT
Providence Medical Center, Portland, OR
Sharp Memorial Hospital, San Diego, CA
Swedish Medical Center, Englewood, CO
The Children's Hospital, Denver, CO
University Hospital, Denver, CO
Veteran's Administration Medical Center, San Diego, CO

1994
Children's Hospital, Denver, CO
Group Health Cooperative of Puget Sound, Seattle, WA
Health One, Inc., Denver, CO
Kaiser Permanente, Oakland, CA
LDS Hospital, Salt Lake City, UT
University Hospital, Denver, CO
Veterans Affairs Medical Center, San Diego, CA

1995
Children's Hospital, Denver, CO
Health One, Inc., Denver, CO
Kaiser Permanente, Anaheim, CA
Kaiser Permanente, Oakland, CA
LDS Hospital, Salt Lake City, UT
Providence Medical Center, Portland, OR
Sharp Healthcare, San Diego, CA
University Hospital, Denver, CO
University Hospital, University of Utah, Salt Lake City, UT
Veterans Affairs Medical Center, San Diego, CA

1996
Kaiser Permanente, Anaheim, CA
Kaiser Permanente, Oakland, CA
Providence Portland Medical Center, OR
The Children's Hospital, Denver, CO
The Medical Center at the University of California San Francisco, CA
Veterans Affairs Medical Center, San Diego, CA

1997
Kaiser Permanente, Oakland, CA
Kaiser Permanente, Pasadena, CA
Providence Portland Medical Center, OR
The Children's Hospital, Denver, CO
University of California Davis Health Systems, CA

1998
Kaiser Permanente, Anaheim, CA
Kaiser Permanente, Oakland, CA
The Children's Hospital, Denver, CO

1999
The Children's Hospital, Denver, CO
Kaiser Permanente, Oakland, CA

2000
Kaiser Permanente, Oakland, CA

2001
Kaiser Permanente, Oakland, CA
Providence Portland Medical Center, OR

2002
Kaiser Permanente, Oakland, CA
Providence Portland Medical Center, OR
The Children's Hospital, Denver, CO

2003
Kaiser Permanente, Oakland, CA

2004
Kaiser Permanente, Oakland, CA
Oregon Health & Science University Hospitals & Clinics, OR

2005
Kaiser Permanente, Oakland, CA

2006
Kaiser Permanente, Oakland, CA
The Children's Hospital, Denver, CO
The Queen's Medical Center, Honolulu, HI
United Medical Center, Cheyenne, WY
University of California San Francisco Medical Center, CA

2007
Lucile Packard Children's Hospital, Palo Alto, CA
Providence Health & Services, OR
The Children's Hospital, Denver, CO
The Queen's Medical Center, Honolulu, HI
University of California San Francisco Medical Center, CA

2008
Lucile Packard Children's Hospital, Palo Alto, CA
University of California San Francisco Medical Center, CA

2009
Alaska Native Medical Center, Anchorage, AK
Banner Good Samaritan Medical Center, Phoenix, AZ
Lucile Packard Children's Hospital at Stanford, Palo Alto, CA
Northern Colorado Medical Center-Banner Health, Greeley, CO
University of California San Francisco Medical Center, CA

2010
Banner Baywood Medical Center, Mesa, AZ
Banner Estrella Medical Center, Phoenix, AZ
Banner Good Samaritan Medical Center, Phoenix, AZ
Banner Health, Arizona and Western Regions, Phoenix, AZ
Banner Heart Hospital, Mesa, AZ
Banner Thunderbird Medical Center, Glendale, AZ
The Children's Hospital, Aurora, CO
Lucile Packard Children's Hospital, Palo Alto, CA
Phoenix Children's Hospital, Phoenix, AZ
University of California San Francisco Medical Center, CA

2011
Banner Health, North Colorado Medical Center, Greeley, CO
Lucile Packard Children's Hospital at Stanford, Palo Alto, CA
Salem Hospital, OR

2012
Lucile Packard Children's Hospital at Stanford, Palo Alto, CA
Oregon Health & Science University Healthcare, Portland, OR
Salem Health, OR
University of California Davis Medical Center, Sacramento, CA

2013
Banner Good Samaritan Medical Center, Phoenix, AZ
Banner Thunderbird Medical Center, Glendale, AZ
Children's Hospital, Aurora, CO
Lucile Packard Children's Hospital at Stanford, Palo Alto, CA
Salem Health, OR
Veterans Administration San Diego Healthcare System, CA

2014
Banner Health, Phoenix, AZ
Children's Hospital, Aurora, CO
Lucile Packard Children's Hospital at Stanford, Palo Alto, CA
Oregon Health & Science University Healthcare, Portland, OR
Providence Health & Services, Renton, WA
Salem Health, OR
University of New Mexico Hospitals, Albuquerque, NM

2015
Children's Hospital Colorado, Aurora, CO
Mayo Clinic, Phoenix, AZ
Providence Health & Services, Renton, WA

2016
Children's Hospital Colorado, Aurora, CO
Hoag Memorial Hospital Presbyterian-Newport Beach, CA
Lucile Packard Children's Hospital, Palo Alto, CA
Mayo Clinic, Phoenix, AZ
Providence Health & Services, Renton, WA
University of California San Francisco Medical Center, CA

2017
Banner Health, Phoenix, AZ
Hoag Memorial Hospital Presbyterian-Newport Beach, CA
Lucile Packard Children's Hospital, Palo Alto, CA
Mayo Clinic, Phoenix, AZ
Providence Health & Services, Renton, WA
University of California San Francisco Medical Center, CA

Clinical Agencies Represented in WAN Presentations:

1994
Marci Catanzaro, Primary Health Care Associates, Seattle, WA
Barbara Trehearne, Group Health Cooperative of Puget Sound, Seattle, WA

1995
Marie J. Driever, Providence Portland Medical Center, Portland, OR
Mary Ann Johnson, Salt Lake Veterans Affairs/University of Utah. UT

1996
Dianne C. Helmer, Lucile Salter Packard Children's Hospital at Stanford, Palo Alto, CA
Mary Ann Johnson, Salt Lake Veterans Affairs/University of Utah, UT

1997
Carol A. Ashton, Intermountain Healthcare, Salt Lake City, UT
Marie J. Driever, Providence Portland Medical Center, Portland, OR

1998
Marci Catanzaro, Primary Health Care Associates, Seattle, WA
Mary Ann Johnson, Salt Lake City, VAMC/GRECC, Utah, UT

1999
Marie Driever, Providence Portland Medical Center, OR
Sheila Quilter Wheeler, TeleTriage Systems, San Anselmo, CA

2000
Diane Brown, Kaiser Permanente East Bay, Walnut Creek, CA
Lowell Wise, Stanford Hospital & Clinics, Palo Alto, CA

2001
Carol Ashton, Health Web Connexions, Salt Lake City, UT
Marie J. Driever, Providence Portland Medical Center, OR

2006
Linda Burnes Bolton, Cedar Sinai Medical Center, Los Angeles, CA
Lori A. Loan, Madigan Army Medical Center, Tacoma, WA

2008
Marilyn P. Chow, Kaiser Permanente, Oakland, CA

2009
Patricia D. Horoho, Madigan Army Medical Center, Tacoma, WA

2010
Anna Gawlinski, UCLA Medical Center, Los Angeles, CA

2014
Mary Anne Mercer, Timor-Leste, Health Alliance International, Seattle, WA
Julia Robinson, Health Alliance International, Seattle, WA

2017
Laura D. Rosenthal, University of Colorado Denver, Aurora, CO

Appendix G
Anna M Shannon Mentorship Award

In 1992, Kathleen Ann Long, former Dean and Professor of the College of Nursing at Montana State University, and Jeanne Kearns, former Executive Director of WIN, established the Anna M. Shannon Mentorship Award. This award recognizes Dr. Shannon, who was Dean and Professor Emeritus of the College of Nursing at Montana State University, for her unselfish efforts to support and promote the professional growth of nurses in the West.

Recipients of the Award

1993	Phyllis Ethridge	Carondelet St. Mary's Hospital, Tucson, AZ
1994	Jeanne Quint Benoliel	University of Washington, Seattle, WA
	Afaf I. Meleis	University of California San Francisco
1995	Ann M. Voda	University of Utah, Salt Lake City, UT
	Helen Nakagawa-Kogan	University of Washington, Seattle, WA
1996	Barbara J. Stewart	Oregon Health Sciences University, Portland, OR
1998	Sheila M. Kodadek	Oregon Health Sciences University, Portland, OR
1999	Joan Kathleen (Kathy) Magilvy	University of Colorado, Denver, CO
2000	Jacquelyn H. Flaskerud	University of California Los Angeles
2001	Jillian Inouye	University of Hawaii at Manoa
2002	Anne Marie Kotzer	The Children's Hospital, Denver, CO
	Nancy White	University of Northern Colorado, Greeley, CO
2003	Clarann Weinert	Montana State University, Bozeman, MT
2004	Julie Fleury	Arizona State University, Tempe, AZ
2005	Mary E. Tiedeman	Brigham Young University, Provo, UT
2006	Noel J. Chrisman	University of Washington, Seattle, WA
	Tina D. DeLapp	University of Alaska, Anchorage, AK
2007	Becky Christian	University of Utah, Salt Lake City, UT
2008	Nancy L. R. Anderson	University of California Los Angeles, CA
2009	Lori A. Loan	Madigan Army Medical Center, Tacoma, WA
2010	Kathryn Records	Arizona State University, Tempe, AZ
2011	Martha J. Lentz	University of Washington, Seattle, WA
2012	Heather M. Young	University of California Davis, Sacramento, CA
2013	Nancy Fugate Woods	University of Washington, Seattle, WA
2014	Terry Badger	University of Arizona, Tucson, AZ
2015	Anne G. Rosenfeld	University of Arizona, Tucson, AZ
2016	Lorraine S. Evangelista	University of California Irvine, CA
2017	Marie L. Lobo	University of New Mexico, Albuquerque, NM

Appendix H
WIN Emeriti

In 1984, the Western Council on Higher Education for Nursing (WCHEN) established the honorary designation of *Emeriti*. It recognizes members, usually retired nurses, who have demonstrated distinguished service to the Western Institute of Nursing or its predecessor, WCHEN.

WIN Emeriti

Carol A. Ashton	Idaho State University
Maxine Atteberry	Loma Linda University
Loretta Hanner Bardewyek	Arizona State University
Marjorie V. Batey	University of Washington
Doris Bloch	DHHS Division of Nursing
Ellamae Branstetter	Arizona State University
Maura Carroll	University of California
Kay Chafey	Montana State University
Thelma Cleveland	Intercollegiate Center for Nursing Education
Pearl Parvin Coulter	University of Arizona
Tina DeLapp	University of Alaska
Marjorie Dunlap	University of California San Francisco
Jo Eleanor Elliott	Division of Nursing
Harold Enarson	Former WICHE Executive Director
Chiyoko Furukawa	University of New Mexico
Barbara Goetz	University of Wyoming
Lulu Wolf Hassenplug	University of California Los Angeles
Beverly Hoeffer	Oregon Health & Science University
Katherine Hoffman	University of Washington
Julie Johnson	CJL Consultants, LLC
Jeanne Kearns	Former WIN Executive Director
Janelle C. Krueger	Arizona State University
Robert Kroepsch	Former WICHE Executive Director
Kathryn Smith Lastreto	University of Colorado
Amelia Leino	University of Wyoming
Martha Lentz	University of Washington
Carol A. Lindeman	Oregon Health & Science University
Joan (Kathy) Magilvy	University of Colorado
Marylou McAthie	Sonoma State University
Beverly B. McCord	University of Arizona
Margaret Metzger	Loretto Heights College
Betty K. Mitsunaga	University of Colorado and University of Washington
Juanita F. Murphy	Arizona State University
Helen Nahm	University of California San Francisco
Ginette A. Pepper	University of Utah
Elda Popiel	University of Colorado
Mildred Quinn	University of Utah
Phillip Sirotkin	Former WICHE Executive Director
Marion M. Schrum	University of Nevada Reno
Anna Shannon	Montana State University

Gladys Sorensen	University of Arizona
Jessie Scott	Division of Nursing
Anna Pearl Sherrick	Montana State University
Bernice Szukalla	Division of Nursing
Ann M. Voda	University of Utah
Verle Waters	Ohlone Community College

Appendix I
Jo Eleanor Elliott Leadership Award

In 1988, Jeanne Kearns established the Jo Eleanor Elliott Leadership Award in honor of Elliott's distinguished service to WCHEN/WIN. Awardees, outstanding leaders, are nominated by two sponsors and selected by a special committee.

Recipients of the Award

1988	Anna Shannon	Montana State University
1989	Ellamae Branstetter	Arizona State University
1990	Jean Lum	University of Hawaii
1991	Carol Lindeman	Oregon Health Sciences University
1992	Marylou McAthie	Sonoma State University
1993	Juanita Murphy	Arizona State University
1994	Elizabeth Nichols	University of Wyoming
1995	Gerry Hansen	Weber State University
1996	Thelma Cleveland	Intercollegiate Center for Nursing Education
1997	Barbara derwinski-Robinson	Montana State University
1998	Jeanne Kearns	Western Institute of Nursing
1999	Marie F. Branch	Former Project Director, WICHE
2000	Helen Ripple	University of California San Francisco Medical Center
2001	Elaine Sorensen Marshall	Brigham Young University
	Pamela H. Mitchell	University of Washington
2002	Tina D. DeLapp	University of Alaska
2003	Jane E. Hirsch	University of California San Francisco Medical Center
2004	Kathleen Chafey	Montana State University
2007	Carol A. Ashton	Idaho State University
	Terry A. Badger	The University of Arizona
2008	Marie J. Driever	Group Health Cooperative, Seattle
2012	Margaret M. Heitkemper	University of Washington
2013	Kathy Magilvy	University of Colorado
2015	Ginette A. Pepper	University of Utah
2017	Judith A. Berg	The University of Arizona

Appendix J
WIN/John A. Hartford Foundation Regional Geriatric Nursing Research Award

In 2001, WIN established the Regional Geriatric Nursing Research Award in partnership with the John A. Hartford Institute for Geriatric Nursing. The purpose of the award is to foster and showcase geriatric nursing research. Two recipients may be selected annually: a senior and a new researcher.

Recipients of the Award

2001	Patricia G. Archbold	Oregon Health & Science University	Senior Researcher
	Linda Phillips	University of Arizona	New Researcher
2002	Jeanie Kayser-Jones	University California San Francisco	Senior Researcher
	Karen A. Talerico	Oregon Health & Science University	New Researcher
2003	Betty L. Chang	University of California Los Angeles	Senior Researcher
	Jill A. Bennett	Oregon Health & Science University	New Researcher
2004	Margaret Dimond	University of Washington	Senior Researcher
	Janet C. Mentes	University of California Los Angeles	New Researcher
2005	Charlene Harrington	University of California San Francisco	Senior Researcher
	Lissi Hansen	Oregon Health & Science University	New Researcher
2006	Julie Fleury	Arizona State University	Senior Researcher
	Nelma Shearer	Arizona State University	New Researcher
2007	Heather M. Young	Oregon Health & Science University	Senior Researcher
	Lynn Woods	University of California Los Angeles	New Researcher
2008	Colleen Keller	Arizona State University	Senior Researcher
	Elena Siegel	Oregon Health & Science University	New Researcher
2009	Ginette A. Pepper	University of Utah	Senior Researcher
	Casey Shillam	University of Portland	New Researcher
2010	Bronwynne Evans	Arizona State University	Senior Researcher
	Glenise L. McKenzie	Oregon Health & Science University	New Researcher
2011	Neva L. Crogan	Washington State University	Senior Researcher
	Debra Bakerjian	University of California Davis	New Researcher
2012	Gloria Adriana Perez	Arizona State University	New Researcher
2013	Janice D. Crist	University of Arizona	Senior Researcher
	Corey G. Nagel	Oregon Health & Science University	New Researcher
2015	Linda S. Edelman	University of Utah	New Researcher
2017	Jane Chung	University of New Mexico	New Researcher

Appendix K
Patsy A. Perry Award for Physiological Nursing Research

In 2005, the first award was given to recognize outstanding biological research conducted by nurses.

Recipients of the Award

2005	Angela Starkweather	Intercollegiate College of Nursing, Washington State University, Spokane, WA
2006	Hilaire J. Thompson	University of Washington
2009	Michael Schlicher	Brooke Army Medical Center, Fort Sam Houston, Texas
2010	Ann Elizabeth Lowe	University of California Los Angeles
2012	Charles A. Downs	Emory University, Atlanta, GA
2013	Lauren Thorngate	University of Washington

Appendix L
Ann M. Voda American Indian/Alaskan Native/First Nation Conference Award

In 2009, the first award was given to support an American Indian/Alaskan Native/First Nation nursing student or clinician to attend the Communicating Nursing Research conference in order to promote nursing student and clinician engagement with the WIN community of scholars and to enhance diversity and networking related to health disparity research, practice, and education.

Recipients of the Award

2009	Molly Butler Aultz	Oregon Health & Science University
2010	Laura Ann Curr Beamer	University of Utah
	David Hodgins	Arizona State University
2011	Rydell (Dale) Todicheeney	University of San Diego
2012	Milissa Grandchamp	Montana State University
2013	Lei-Lani White	Arizona State University
2014	Michelle Kahn-John	University of Colorado
2016	Nicholas L. Zumwalt	University of Arizona
2017	Lenora Duncan Littledeer	University of New Mexico

Appendix M
WIN/John A. Hartford Foundation Regional Geriatric Nursing Education Award

In 2011, WIN partnered with the John A. Hartford Foundation to provide the Regional Nursing Education Award. The funds for the award are offered by the OHSU Hartford Center.

Recipients of the Award

2012	Catherine Van Son	Washington State University
2013	Glenise McKenzie	Oregon Health & Science University
2014	Young-Shin Lee	San Diego State University

Appendix N

Communicating Nursing Research Conference Participants & Presentations

Year	Total Papers	Podium Presentations	Symposia	Posters	Research Information Exchange
1968	5	5 (+5 critique)			
1969	5	5 (+6 critique)			
1970	6	6 (+5 critique)			
1971	6	6 (+6 critique)			
1972	9	9 (+9 critique)			
1973	13	13 (+7 critique)			
1974	13	13 (+11 critique)			
1975	26	26 (+2 critique) (+8 discussion)			
1976	30	30 (+4 discussion)			
1977	17	17 (+8 discussion)			
1978	56	17	7	29	
1979		18	8	25	
1980		19	5	29	
1981		29	3	21	
1982		57	11	9	
1983	62	32	7	11	
1984	88	52	8	14	71
1985		55	8	30	61
1986		53	8	20	75
1987	128	74	12	30	91
1988	86	62	5	33	107
1989	124	68	11	34	127
1990	159	97	13	47	134
1991	126	79	11	38	36
1992	127	71	13	47	119
1993	163	85	18	24	64
1994	128	71	13	25	81
1995	110	74	9	24	77
1996	64	47	4	26	65
1997	96	64	8	33	64
1998	97	52	10	35	56
1999	93	43	10	30	55
2000	100	49	10	44	37
2001	159	57	20	80	26
2002	159	68	18	94	24
2003	164	58	22	103	31
2004	156	93	19	127	60
2005	168	86	16	141	73
2006	134	79	10	128	81
2007	200	108	18	128	82
2008	166	82	17	187	81
2009	178	101	15	182	105
2010	220	123	19	194	130
2011	185	86	20	220	132
2012	224	117	21	306	116
2013	239	117	24	428	166
2014	240	107	24	454	175
2015	208	128	17	371	126
2016	194	130	14	465	226

WCHEN/WIN ADMINISTRATIVE STAFF

Jo Eleanor Elliot
1957-1980	Director, WICHE Nursing Programs
	Nurse Consultant
	Executive Secretary, WCHEN

Jeanne Kearns
1975-1980	Associate Director, WICHE Nursing Programs
1980-1981	Acting Director, WICHE Nursing Programs
	Executive Secretary, WCHEN
1982-1985	Director, WICHE Nursing Programs
	Executive Secretary WCHEN
1986-1996	Executive Director, WIN

Sally Ruybal
1981-1982	Director, WICHE Nursing Programs
	Executive Secretary, WCHEN

Patricia Uris
1987-1990	Associate Director, WIN

Paula McNeil
1996 –	Executive Director, WIN
2004 -	Project Director, NEXus

Anna Galas
2006 -	Project Coordinator/Manager, NEXus

Bo Perry
2010 -	Conference Manager

WCHEN/WIN ADMINISTRATIVE SUPPORT STAFF

1950s	1990s
Jean Davis	Kay Groeneveld
	H. Don Harper
1960s	Jane Innes
Jean Davis	Jami Switzer
1970s	2000s
Jon Bunnell	Lana Kamerer
Leah Goedert	Melissa Hill
Elizabeth Sharp	Hillary Panzer
Mary Sue Watkins	Diane Anderson, NEXus
Brenda Yearwood	Ashley Branch, NEXus
	2010s
1980s	Leah Brandis, NEXus
Dianne Bernier	Kate Higgins
Cecilia Graber	Laura Hottman
Marla Hamby	
Jane E. Innes	
Anita Pearce	

WCHEN/WIN STAFF FOR PROJECTS, CONTRACTS OR SURVEYS

1950s

Jo Eleanor Elliott
Regional Conference on Research in Nursing
Continuing Education for Leadership
Reports on Research Conducted by Faculty
Nurses for the West
Defining Clinical Content: Graduate Nursing Program

1960s

Marjorie Batey
Developing a Q-Sort Instrument to Delineate Differences between Graduates of
Baccalaureate and Associates Degree Programs
Regional Conferences on Research in Nursing
Jo Eleanor Elliott
Staff Development Workshop for Nursing Directors
Improving Instruction through the Use of Selected Tools and Technologies
One Approach to the Identification of Essential Content in Baccalaureate
Programs in Nursing
Today and Tomorrow in Western Nursing
Roma Blasche
Curriculum, Improvement Project
Sally Lazar
Continuing Education in Psychiatric Mental Health for Faculty in Associate
Degree Programs
Nona Tiller Pair
Coordinator, Special Nursing Projects
Juereta Smith
Curriculum Improvement Project

1970s

Violet Archuleta
Training Nurses to Improve Patient Education
Jeanne Berthold
Regional Program for Nursing Research and Development
Marie Branch
Faculty Development to Meet Minority Group Needs: Recruitment, Retention
and Curriculum Change
Models for Introducing Cultural Diversity in Nursing Curricula
Rosemary Campos
Regional Program for Nursing Research and Development
Jo Eleanor Elliott
Analysis and Planning for Improved Distribution of Nursing Personnel and Services
Mark Fetler
Compilation of Nursing Research Instruments
Jeanne Kearns
Analysis and Planning for Improved Distribution of Nursing Personnel and
Services
Continuing Education Projects for Nurses – Idaho, Montana, Wyoming
Training Nurses to Improve Patient Education

Sheila Kodadek
Continuing Education in Psychiatric Mental Health Nursing for Faculty in
Associate Degree Programs
Analysis and Planning for Improved Distribution of Nursing Personnel and Services
Janelle Kruger
Regional Program for Nursing Research and Development
Carol Lindeman
Regional Program for Nursing Research and Development
Analysis and Planning for Improved Distribution of Nursing Personnel and Services
Doreen Maher
Training Nurses to Improve Patient Education
Patricia McAtee
Development of Nurse Faculty for Improving and Expanding Continuing
Education and Inservice Education Programs
Sharon Morgan
Compilation of Nursing Research Instruments
Allen Nelson
Regional Program for Nursing Research and Development
Ora Plummer
Training Nurses to Improve Patient Education
Mary Jane Ward
Compilation of Nursing Research Instruments
Carmen Westwick
Feasibility Study: Leadership Preparation for Complex Organization

Kathy Allman   Jean L. J. Lum
Paul Athey   Kevin Mactavish
Esther Bright   David Makowski
Jon Bunnell   Kenneth Malanowicz
Erin Cannon   Irene Munoz
Christina Caramana   Elda Popiel
Douglas Collier   Ken Saucer
Renda Dale   Mary Segall
Jo Eleanor Elliott   Mark Smith
Pauline Gingras   Gwen Thorton
Rob Gray   Ken Traut
William Johnston   Chris Veasey
Wayne Kirschling   Ken Woellhof
Gregory Leonhard
Analysis and Planning for Improved Distribution of Nursing Personnel and Services

1980s
Karen Babich
Continuing Education to Improve Mental Health
Linda Brown
Compilation of Nursing Research Instruments
Carol Burckhardt
Compilation of Nursing Research Instruments
Frank Javorick
Changing Nurses' Participation in Health Planning

1990s

Jeanne Kearns
  Nursing Continuing Education Program: Special Needs of Racial/Ethnic Minority Populations who Abuse Alcohol and Other Drugs
  Dissemination of Information Related to Strengthening of Nursing Education and Practice and to Set Future Directions
Paula McNeil
  Improving Healthcare through Nursing Informatics

2000s

Paula McNeil
  The Nursing Education Xchange: Partnering to Increase the Capacity of Nursing PhD Programs, US Department of Education (P116B040822); US Department of Health and Human Services, Health Resources and Services Administration (D09HP09070).
Anna Galas
  The Nursing Education Xchange: Partnering to Increase the Capacity of Nursing PhD Programs, US Department of Education (P116B040822); US Department of Health and Human Services, Health Resources and Services Administration (D09HP09070).

WCHEN/WIN SUPPORT STAFF FOR PROJECTS, CONTRACTS OR SURVEYS
1950s

Christine Rose	Dorothy Torgerson
Jean Davis	

1960s

Joyce Engle	Maxine Reeves
Gail Kuse	Linda Van Dyke

1970s

Teresa Baca	Connie Martino-Huebner
Judith Bay	Cheryl McLean
Cheryl Bishop	Karen Miller
Alice Bowden	Edith Modafferi
Renee Browning	Connie Murphy
Joan Byers	Patty Nettles
Helen Calvo	Violet Nielson
Gloria Edwards	Betty Jean Oden
Karen Ellsworth	Anita Pearce
Ruth French	Judy Proges
Maureen Gamble	George Rannie
Dee Girolamo	Pat Riley
Jean Gribble	Paula Rosen
Margot Griffith	Ellen Schneider
Barbara Hardesty	Betty Scott
Sandra Hays	Mary Shapek

Connie Huebner
Sharon Lane
Kay Lindsey
Eileen Maresca
Dianna Martinez

Roma Simons
Kay Vaughn
Eileen Volkman
Linda Wanamaker
Jacqueline Ware

1980s
Nancy Baskett
Brenda Brittain
Elsa Garcia
Jill Goldwater
Cecilia Graeber
Marla Hamby

Louise Lawrence
Cheryl McLean
Dorothy Read
Margaret Timothy
Norma Walker

1990s
Kay Groeneveld

Mary Beth Tyler

2000s
E. Dianne Anderson
Ashley Branch

Anna Galas